# The Ideal Diet For Health

## A Pesco-Mediterranean Diet with Intermittent Fasting: Get Your Natural Weight for Life

Xavier Vega

contained within this document, including, but not limited to, errors, omissions, or inaccuracies.

# Table of Contents

# Finding The Ideal Diet

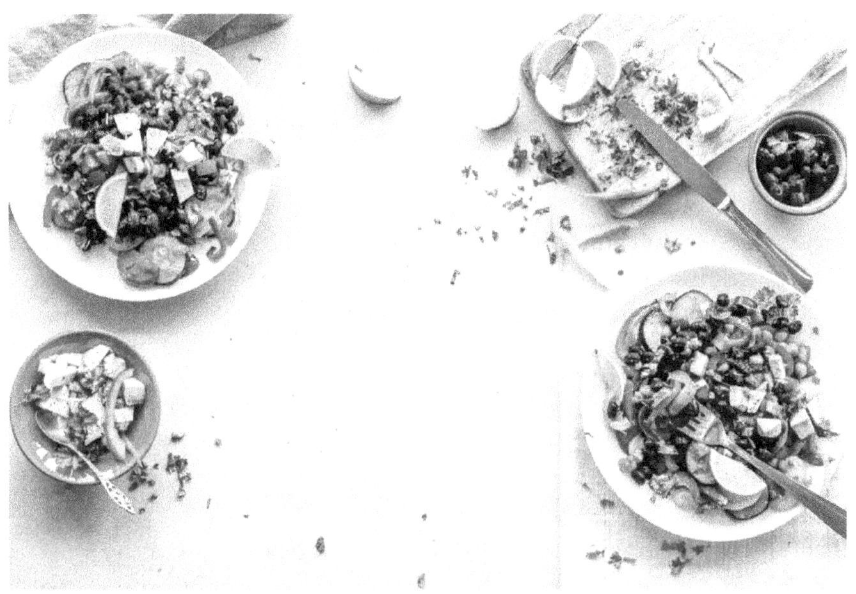

Have you ever wondered about the 'perfect' diet?

Unfortunately, there is no such thing. But there is an 'ideal' diet for health, which is what this book is all about. Human beings are considered "opportunistic omnivores." This means that through evolution, our bodies have adapted to get our nutrients and calories from animal and plant food sources. Even our earliest ancestors lived on fruits they foraged and animals they hunted. Until now, most humans (with the exception of those who have chosen to follow a purely plant-based diet) survive and thrive on one type of omnivorous diet or another.

While consuming both plants and animals is considered 'normal,' it isn't always healthy. Nowadays, a lot of people tend to focus too much on animal products to the point of overconsumption. The worst part is, the animal products being chosen are processed meat products instead of fresh meat. Processed meat products such as hotdogs, bacon, and deli meats are high in chemical additives, saturated fats, and other unhealthy ingredients. If you're fond of processed meats (and other processed animal-based products), you may want to change your diet now—and since you're reading this book, it means you are already interested in making a change for the better. Good for you!

Plant-based diets such as veganism and vegetarianism seem like healthy diets too. And they are... if followed correctly. But following these diets too strictly or not following them correctly can cause a number of adverse side effects too, the most dangerous of which are nutrient deficiencies. If left unchecked or untreated, these deficiencies can increase the risk of developing conditions like anemia, sarcopenia, and osteopenia, for example. Although many people thrive on plant-based diets, this doesn't mean that such diets are ideal.

So... what is the ideal diet?

When you think about it, the most logical and healthiest compromise is to combine a diet that is rich in plants with healthy animal food sources, mainly fish and seafood. Yes, there is such a diet and even though it's relatively new, it is already growing in popularity as more experts are discovering the amazing potential of this diet. I am talking about the Pesco-Mediterranean diet, which is a combination of the Pescatarian diet and the Mediterranean diet, one of the healthiest diets in the world. Clinical trials and studies conducted about the Pesco-Mediterranean diet have shown that this is the ideal diet for improving cardiovascular health. But this isn't the only benefit. There are many more. The foundation of the Pesco-Mediterranean diet is fruits, veggies, legumes, nuts, seeds, whole grains, fermented dairy products, olive oil, fish, and seafood. In terms of beverages, the best options are plain tea, coffee, and, of course, water.

In itself, this diet already has a lot of potential. But we will be taking things a step further as you will learn how to combine this with intermittent fasting too. Being a relatively new diet (although the Pescatarian and Mediterranean diets have been around for some time already), there is much to learn about the Pesco-Mediterranean diet. In this book, you will learn all of the fundamentals of this diet to help you understand why it is being touted as the ideal diet for health.

But before we continue, let me share my story with you. When learning new things, it is always more beneficial to understand your source, which, in this case, is me. I am Xavier Vega, a writer who is always inspired to craft educational content that focuses on sports, healthy lifestyles, and healthy food, among others. I have always had an interest in the fields of personal development, healthy nutrition, and longevity. But I was not always like this. For a very long time, I struggled with smoking addiction and alcoholism. These unhealthy habits were such a big part of my life that I didn't think I could get rid of them.

But I did.

At one point, I decided to turn my life around by fighting my addictions. It wasn't an easy journey but it was fulfilling. For years, I devoted myself to quitting these habits—smoking and alcohol—by working out and following a healthy diet. Through patience, hard work, and a lot of self-kindness, I transformed my life into a healthier and more meaningful one.

Because I was able to successfully pull myself out of the unhealthy life I used to live, I have then decided to dedicate my life to helping others fight addictions too. I try my best to inspire and encourage those around me to live a healthier life by exercising regularly and making healthier food choices. Now, when I am not writing, I enjoy reading books, especially on health and nutrition. I also engage in different sports and outdoor activities, I cook my own nutritious meals, and I spend a lot of time at the gym. These are the habits I had learned throughout my journey. Habits that I want to share with others.

In my first book entitled, "Mind Killer," I focused on addiction. In that book, I focused on how to stop drinking and changing one's life by gaining freedom and health. I delved into the different types of addiction, the wonders of incorporating sports into one's life, and healthy eating. My first book also included a guide on how to gain one's freedom and mental well-being while maintaining emotional stability. If you're interested in all of these things, you may want to check it out!

But let's get back to this book. As an expert in health and nutrition, I have already helped a hundred people to fight addiction, clean up their lives, and live happier, more fulfilled lives. I believe that everyone has what it takes to turn their life around—even you. If you're looking for an ideal diet to follow, now is the time to learn about it. By the end of this book, you will understand what this diet is all about, why you need to start following it, and how to follow it. If you're ready to take a meaningful journey to improve your health through your diet, let's begin!

# Chapter 1:

# The Amazing Diet Combination

The world of health and diets has always been interesting because of all the diet trends that have emerged in recent years. All of these diets have their own benefits and downsides. More and more people are starting to show more interest in their health, which is why these diets have become wildly popular. However, we have yet to see the 'perfect' diet that offers only benefits without any risks. Right now, such a diet doesn't exist yet, but there is one that comes pretty close—the Pesco-Mediterranean diet.

This diet is ideal for reducing your risk of cardiovascular disease, losing weight, and improving your overall health. It focuses on plant-based foods but it also includes healthy animal-based food sources to ensure that you get all of the nutrients you need to stay healthy. This diet is a combination of two healthy diets—pescatarian and Mediterranean—both of which offer their own set of health benefits. When combined, they create a wonderfully nutrient-dense, simple diet that you will surely love. And when you combine this with intermittent fasting, you can get even more health benefits. We will discuss this further later. For now, let's focus on the basics of the diet to help you understand it better.

# All About the Pescatarian Diet

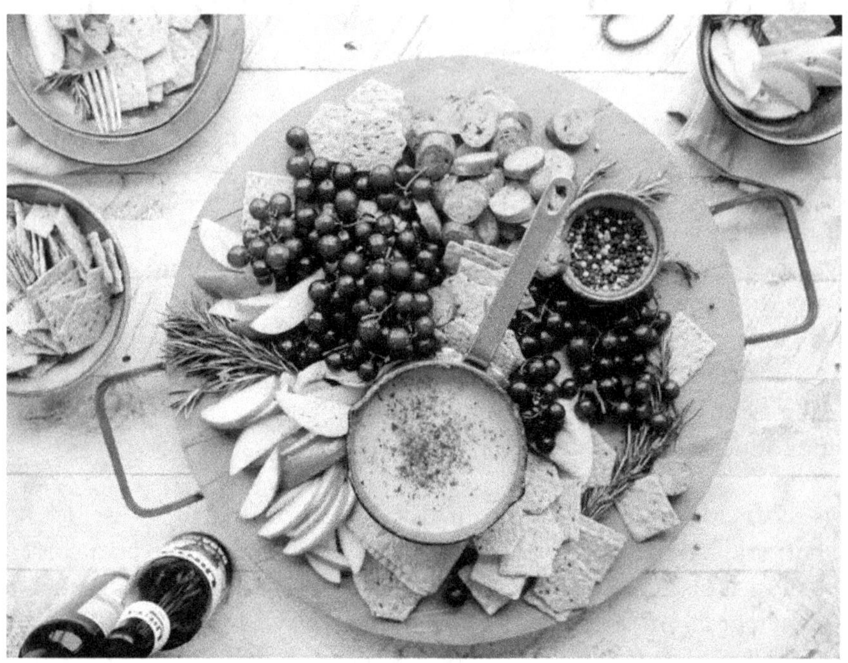

If you try to compare the healthiest diets in the world, you will realize that fish is one of the main foods. This makes the pescatarian diet fit right into this category since the term 'pesce' means fish. The pescatarian diet focuses on fish and other types of seafood as the main source of protein. This is a very simple diet and it's flexible enough to allow you to continue eating your favorite foods. As a pescatarian, you can even include dairy and eggs in your diet, as long as you consume these moderately.

Although the pescatarian diet focuses on fish, it's not an all-fish and seafood diet. Typically, you just have to make sure that you eat a minimum of two or more fish or seafood meals each week. For the rest of your meals and snacks, you would focus on plant-based food sources. This part of the diet makes it similar to the Mediterranean diet, which is why these diets work so well together. This diet doesn't come with strict guidelines nor will it make you feel restricted either. You can even combine this diet with other types of diets too.

Most people who follow the pescatarian diet are health conscious and tend to be very mindful when it comes to planning their meals. For instance, people who want to become vegetarians but aren't ready to give up meat completely yet may start by following the pescatarian diet. This diet is also ideal for people who want to give up red meat but don't want to shift to a diet that is completely plant-based. Either way, transitioning to the pescatarian diet comes with a host of health benefits making it an amazing diet to follow. Mainly, this diet offers anti-inflammatory benefits while promoting cardiovascular health. By following this diet, you can reduce your risk of developing chronic diseases like arthritis, type 2 diabetes, and heart disease, for example.

Aside from health benefits, some people also follow this diet for ethical and environmental reasons. Generally, fish and seafood have a smaller carbon footprint compared to poultry or livestock. Although there are still concerns in terms of overfishing and the efficiency of fuel used for fishing boats, making smarter choices when purchasing fish can help reduce or avoid such concerns.

Of course, the pescatarian diet is not perfect. It has huge potential for providing health benefits but if it's not followed properly, you shouldn't expect these benefits to take effect any time soon. For instance, if you choose to cut out red meat in an attempt to follow this diet but you increase your intake of unhealthy and processed plant-based food sources, you won't be doing your body good. The pescatarian diet isn't strict but this doesn't mean that you can eat anything you want while on it. Even when it comes to fish, there are better choices to opt for if you want to stay healthy. To improve your health, it's best to focus on fatty fish like tuna, salmon, and mackerel, for example. This is because such fish varieties offer more omega-3s compared to others. So you need to plan your meals carefully to make sure that you're giving yourself the best version of the pescatarian diet possible.

Since the pescatarian diet is well-rounded, it can potentially supply you with all of the nutrition you need each day. Plants, fish, and seafood are enough to help you avoid nutrient deficiencies. Because of this, most people who follow the diet don't have to take supplements along with it. Of course, if you want to make sure, you can ask your doctor about it. Talk to your doctor about the pescatarian diet and even present them with a sample meal plan. This information will make it easier for your doctor to determine whether you need to take supplements or not.

## All About the Mediterranean Diet

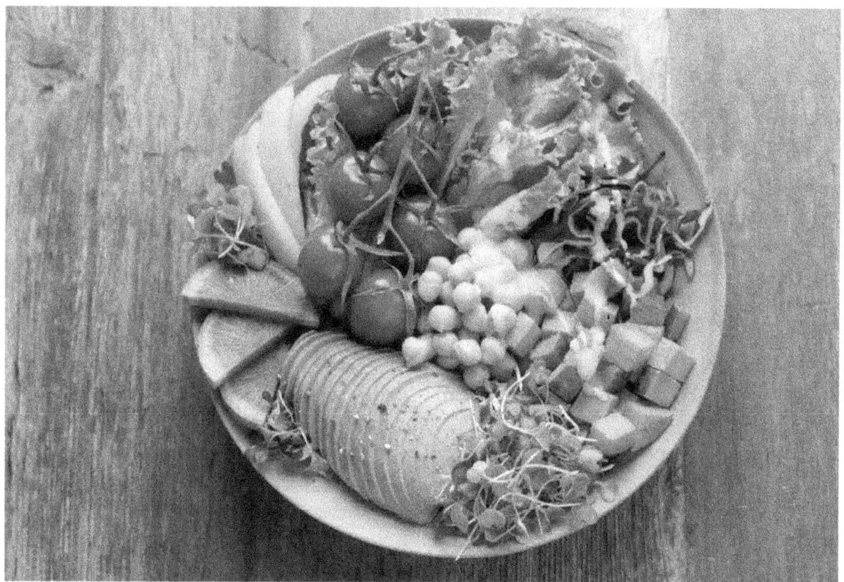

The Mediterranean diet focuses on traditional foods consumed by people in Greece and other countries in the Mediterranean region. It focuses on fruits, vegetables, fish, olive oil, and whole grains, all of which are rich in nutrients. Since this diet has been around for some time now, it has been studied by many researchers and medical experts. Based on these studies, the Mediterranean diet can help reduce the risk of diabetes, heart disease, and other health conditions including cancer. This diet is more of an eating pattern that encourages you to eat whole foods, add variety to your diet, and enjoy flavorful meals. Just like the pescatarian diet, it doesn't involve strict restriction, which is why it is highly sustainable.

Those who follow the Mediterranean diet love it because the dishes eaten are so simple and flavorful. The ingredients used for these meals are sustainable, easy to find, and extremely healthy. This diet first became public in the 1970s by Ancel Keys, a scientist who is most famous for the "Seven Countries Study," wherein he examined the connection between heart disease rates and the intake of dietary fat. Although this study has undergone a lot of criticism over the years, it still has some significant takeaways. For one, this study identifies that the people who lived in Greece, specifically the Crete Region had lower heart disease rates despite having high rates of overall fat intake. Based on these facts, Keys believed that the eating style of these people—the Mediterranean diet—was largely responsible for this.

But during that time, people in the US didn't embrace the Mediterranean diet yet. It was only in the year 1993 when a non-profit organization known as Oldways partnered up with the World Health Organization, and the Harvard School of Public Health to come up with a diet pyramid based on the Mediterranean diet. This pyramid became the alternative to the food pyramid of the USDA and it focused on foods from the Mediterranean region. It also emphasized the importance of social connections and physical activity.

Since then, interest in the diet was awakened. In the 1960s, when experts realized that Greece, Italy, and other countries in the Mediterranean region had fewer deaths caused by coronary heart disease, they started studying the diet more. This is when they discovered that the diet is associated with a reduced risk of cardiovascular disease and other health conditions. Now, the Mediterranean diet is considered one of the healthiest eating plans that promotes health while preventing chronic diseases. The World Health Organization also considers this as a highly sustainable eating pattern that can be followed long-term.

The dietary recommendations for the Mediterranean diet are similar to the pescatarian diet. It mainly consists of fruits, vegetables, whole grains, nuts, seeds, olive oil, fish, and other healthy fats. You can also have eggs on this diet. But the difference is, this diet allows minimal amounts of red and white meat. It also allows you to enjoy red wine in moderation. After all, meals are much more enjoyable with a glass of red wine now and then.

Just like the pescatarian diet, the Mediterranean diet is based on plant-based food sources instead of meat-based food sources. It also encourages physical activity and sharing your meals with friends and family. In other words, it is more holistic as it focuses on other aspects, not just your diet. If you plan to follow the Pesco-Mediterranean diet, you can start by following either of these diets first. Just remember that your long-term goal is to combine these diets to create a sustainable dietary lifestyle that will allow you to maintain your health.

# The Pesco-Mediterranean Diet: A Perfect Combination

Now that you know all about the pescatarian diet and the Mediterranean diet, it's time to combine them to create something special. Since these diets have a lot of similarities, it's easy to put them together to come up with an easy to follow, scrumptious, and healthy way of eating. By combining these diets, you will also be combining the potential health benefits they have to offer. Many clinical trials and epidemiological studies have shown the effectiveness of these diets in improving health. Because of their very nature, these diets will help you learn how to focus on healthier food options without feeling like you are restricting or depriving yourself of "good food."

One of the best things about the Pesco-Mediterranean diet is the ease by which you can follow it. As long as you know what foods to focus on and what foods to gradually wean yourself off of (don't worry, this list isn't very long), you will discover how natural this diet feels and how beneficial it is to your life. Just like the pescatarian and Mediterranean diets, the Pesco-Mediterranean diet is plant-rich while allowing the consumption of meat too—mainly fish and seafood. It also encourages the consumption of healthy fats to make all of your dishes more flavorful and satisfying. And as soon as you understand what the diet involves, transitioning into it will become a positive and enjoyable experience for you. After some time, you can start reaping the benefits of the best dietary decision you can make for yourself.

# Chapter 2

# All About the Pesco-Mediterranean Diet

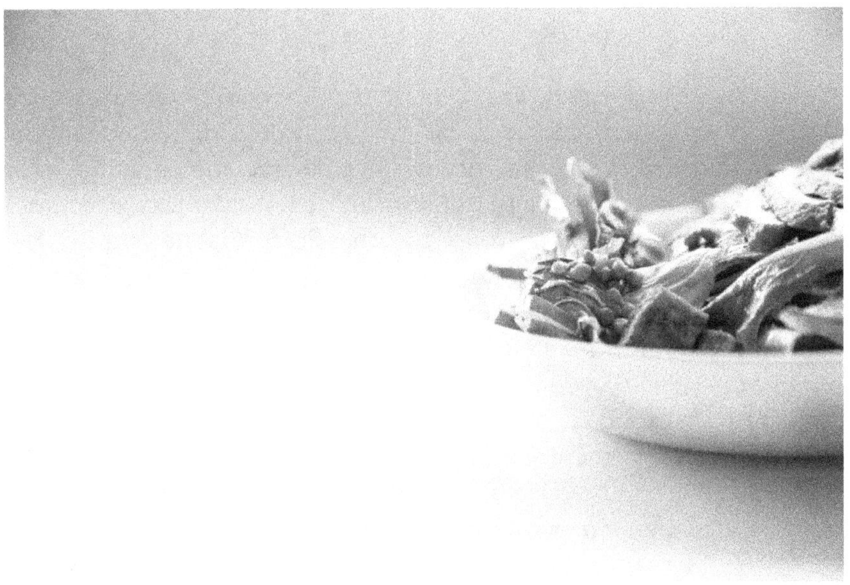

The Pesco-Mediterranean diet is rich in whole grains, plants, seeds, nuts, extra-virgin olive oil, other types of healthy fats, fish, and seafood. This is the ideal diet to improve your cardiovascular health and other aspects of your health too. Even though human beings are omnivores and we can survive on different types of foods, most people still struggle with their diets. In fact, the struggle to find the perfect diet has been going on for centuries, which is why so many diets have emerged over the years.

When it comes to diets, those which are rich in plants seem to be more popular and sustainable because of the health benefits they offer. But a diet that is purely plant-based isn't always the ideal diet for most people, especially in modern Western cultures. In America, for instance, many people prefer diets that are high in meat and other animal-based food sources. Unfortunately, if you start focusing on highly-processed animal products that are readily available and highly convenient, that's when you start experiencing issues with your health. The good news is that the Pesco-Mediterranean diet can be your solution to the dilemma of omnivores. Instead of completely giving up animals or plants, you can enjoy both without compromising your health.

So many studies, research, and clinical trials have supported the fact that fish is an essential part of any heart-healthy diet. In fact, the Dietary Guidelines for Americans include recommendations for consuming fish instead of eggs, poultry, and red meat at least two times each week. When you start following the Pesco-Mediterranean diet, you will be focusing on fish and seafood as your main protein source, which means that you will gradually minimize your consumption of poultry and red meat. Naturally, this means that you will be improving the nutrition value of your diet as you increase your fish intake along with plant-based foods too. Aside from this, the Pesco-Mediterranean diet also encourages the use of extra-virgin olive oil and other healthy fats instead of using butter, corn oil, palm oil, or any other processed oils that don't do anything good for your health.

While following this diet, you would have to pay special attention to extra-virgin olive oil as this is the unrefined, higher-quality version of olive oil (which is also a good option). Because of this, it offers cardiometabolic benefits like increasing your good cholesterol levels and reducing your levels of bad cholesterol. This type of oil makes your dishes richer and more flavorful while adding more fiber and healthy fats to your dishes. For a lot of people, one of the best things about the Pesco-Mediterranean diet is that it allows eggs and dairy products. Although this doesn't mean that you should indulge in hard cheese, butter, and other dairy products that contain a lot of salt and saturated fats. When it comes to dairy, you need to be very picky, especially if you want to get the most out of this unique diet. As for eggs, these can be an excellent substitute for red meat along with fish and seafood.

As you will soon come to discover, this diet is so simple that it won't take much effort from you to follow. Even if you rely heavily on processed foods, it will be easy to transition into the Pesco-Mediterranean diet simply because it focuses on foods that are nutrient-dense, satisfying, and delicious. You may need some time to get used to it but your body will definitely thank you for this change.

## How Does It Work?

If you tried to create an ideal diet that will improve the health of your heart, help you lose weight, and provide other benefits to your health, the diet you will come up with will probably look a lot like the Pesco-Mediterranean diet. This is a plant-rich diet flavored with olive oil and other healthy fats then enriched with fish and seafood. What more can you ask for?

This type of eating style has a lot of benefits, especially in the long-term. It works to improve your health by providing your body with clean, natural, and essential nutrients from all of the foods you will be eating while following the diet. Unlike the Standard American Diet and other Western eating habits, this diet doesn't include unhealthy foods like refined carbs, saturated fat, and processed food products. It's also more beneficial than diets that are purely plant-based because animal food sources will help reduce the risk of developing anemia, weak bones, weak muscles, or nutrient deficiencies. The best part is, this diet is delicious, satiating, and highly sustainable making it a perfect choice whether you are at the peak of your health or you want to overcome certain health issues.

Experts have given the traditional Mediterranean diet the title of, "The Gold Standard for Cardiovascular Health." To enjoy this main benefit and all others the diet has to over (combined with the benefits of the pescatarian diet), you can start making small changes to your diet. As with any other diet, you don't have to dive into the Pesco-Mediterranean diet in a day, especially if this diet is very far from what you are used to. Instead, you should create a plan for how you will start on the diet and continue following it until you have transitioned fully. For instance, instead of eating meat every day of the week, replace one or two days with fish or seafood dishes. Once or twice a week, try to consume plant-based meals that include your favorite veggies. Taking these small steps will make it easier for you to change your diet while giving your body time to adjust as well. This strategy will also help you feel more positive about the diet since you won't feel like you are restricting yourself from eating meat and other foods that don't belong to the Pesco-Mediterranean diet.

As you make these changes, your body will already start feeling the good effects of the healthy foods you eat. Since the foods on this diet are filled with vitamins, minerals, antioxidants, and other nutrients, good changes will occur within your body and soon, you will start feeling yourself getting stronger, healthier, and more energized. Simple as this diet might seem, it is extremely effective. And this is why it's considered the ideal diet for health.

## What Science Has To Say

If you are like me and all other people who have started reading about a diet that can potentially improve their health, you would like to know if the diet has been studied by experts in the field. Studies, research, and clinical trials are very important as these can either contradict or support anecdotal evidence coming from the followers of a certain diet—in this case, the Pesco-Mediterranean diet. The good news is, this diet has already been the focus of studies. Both the pescatarian and Mediterranean diets have been the focus of many studies, which is why both diets have their own followings.

One study conducted about the Mediterranean diet showed that this diet helps reduce the risk of cardiovascular events (Estruch, R., et. al., 2013). This effect came from the reduced levels of LDL ('bad') cholesterol levels in those who followed the diet. In another study, researchers discovered that the Mediterranean diet can also help those who suffer from type 2 diabetes (Salas-Salvado, J., et. al., 2010). According to this study, the diet can help prevent type 2 diabetes, especially in those who have a high risk of cardiovascular disease. Yet another study showed that this traditional diet can help reduce the prevalence of metabolic syndrome along with the cardiovascular risk that is typically associated with MS (Esposito, K. et. al., 2004). According to the study, this benefit mainly comes from the anti-inflammatory benefits that the foods in the diet offer. These are just some examples of studies conducted about this simple yet unbelievably healthy diet. There are many more.

As for the pescatarian diet, there are many studies done about it too. One such study showed that there is a link between this diet (and other plant-based diets) and a reduced risk of ischaemic heart disease (Mahase, E., 2019). These results were compared to those who follow diets that include a lot of meat. In another study, the researchers discovered that the pescatarian diet along with the vegetarian and flexitarian diet can help improve one's cardiovascular risk profile (Wozniak, H., et. al., 2020). The participants who followed these studies also had lower cholesterol levels, reduced risk of hypertension, and lower BMI too. As you can see, the benefits of the pescatarian and Mediterranean diets are quite similar since the diets themselves are similar too.

So... Do the same benefits apply when these diets are put together?

For the Pesco-Mediterranean diet, the most significant study conducted about it focused on heart health and combining this diet with intermittent fasting (O' Keefe, J., et. al., 2020). In this study, the researchers examined the effects of the Pesco-Mediterranean diet to health. A massive review was conducted based on the available data and they concluded that the diet is ideal for the optimization of cardiovascular health. By following this diet, you can protect your heart from stroke, clogged blood vessels, heart attack, and even other health issues like dementia.

The heart-healthy benefits of the Pesco-Mediterranean diet are even more potent than those of other plant-based diets like vegan, semi-vegetarian, or lacto-ovo vegetarian diets. According to this study, this is largely because of the focus on fatty fish that are rich in omega-3s. These are the main components that reduce the risk of heart disease. Combining these effects with the anti-inflammatory benefits of plants and the elimination of processed food products and red meat gives you a super-powered eating plan that supports your overall health.

With all of these studies and more, it's obvious that the Pesco-Mediterranean diet is the one to look out for. Although the studies focused on this diet aren't as numerous as those of other diets, the fact that this diet is becoming more popular already serves as a "go signal" for researchers and health experts to focus more on it. For now, the few studies about the Pesco-Mediterranean diet are showing promising results and if you want to stay updated, you can continue your research after learning more about this super style of eating.

# Chapter 3: How to Start on the Pesco-Mediterranean Diet

The Pesco-Mediterranean diet is rich in plants, whole grains, nuts, seeds, fish, seafood, and healthy fats like extra-virgin olive oil. Since this diet is very simple, it's extremely easy to follow, especially since it doesn't focus on caloric restriction or severely limiting yourself from eating certain types of foods. Instead, this diet will help you learn how to become a healthier eater in the long-run. This is more beneficial for you as there is a higher likelihood that you will always make healthy food choices when you see how delicious and satisfying healthy foods are and how these foods improve your health from the inside.

# What to Eat

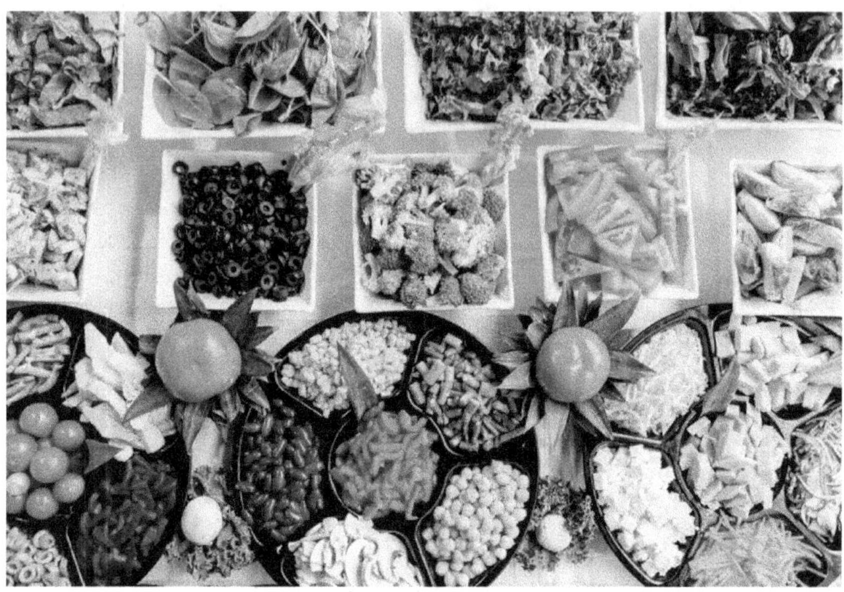

By now, you should already know that the Pesco-Mediterranean diet isn't rigid. It is flexible enough to help you learn how to eat healthily while still allowing you to have a 'treat' once in a while. For instance, some diets require you to give up certain food groups to make sure that the diets work. But here, you would generally have to avoid certain foods like poultry and meat, for instance, but if you're at a party or you're sharing a meal with your family, you don't have to restrict yourself from having a serving of chicken or beef.

This is because the Pesco-Mediterranean diet is more about encouraging yourself to make better dietary choices in the long-run. Since it doesn't focus on restriction, this diet is a lot easier to follow and sustain. That being said, there are certain foods that are recommended on this diet to ensure that you enjoy all the potential benefits it has to offer. Both the pescatarian and Mediterranean diets are based on fruits, veggies, whole grains, nuts, fish, and seafood, this makes them work together perfectly. To make things easier for you, here are the foods to eat on the Pesco-Mediterranean diet:

- **Fish and Seafood**

While on the Pesco-Mediterranean diet, your main animal sources would be fish and seafood. These foods contain different kinds of vitamins, minerals, and essential nutrients making them a better source of protein than red meat and poultry. When choosing fish and seafood from your diet,

- Freshwater fish like perch, trout, bluegill, catfish, tilapia, pollock, bass, and walleye.
- Saltwater fish like tuna, mackerel, herring, salmon, and sardines.
- Seafood like oysters, clams, shrimp, crabs, lobsters, scallops, and mussels.
- Canned fish like sardines, salmon, and tuna.
- Frozen fish and seafood like salmon, trout, shrimp, and herring.

- **Fruits and Vegetables**

Since this diet focuses more on plant-based foods, fruits and veggies are a huge part of it. A typical meal on this diet consists of veggies, whole grain, complex carbs, and a fish or seafood protein (sometimes a plant protein). Then it can include a piece of fruit to add some sweetness and nutrition to the meal. For this diet, there are no limitations in terms of the types of fruits and veggies you can have. To make the most of the Pesco-Mediterranean diet, you should familiarize yourself with all the fruits and veggies with the colors of the rainbow.

- **Healthy Fats and Oils**

Fat is an important part of your diet so you shouldn't be scared of it. Unfortunately, many diets claim that fats are unhealthy and they prevent you from losing weight. But the fact is, adding healthy fats to your diet will make you healthier while making your diet richer and more flavorful. Fats and oils supply your body with essential fats and calories to aid in the absorption of fat-soluble vitamins like vitamin A, vitamin D, vitamin E, and vitamin K. On this diet, the main focus should be on olive oil and extra-virgin olive oil but you can also enjoy other oils such as sunflower, avocado, or canola oils, for example when cooking meals, making salad dressings, and so on.

- **Herbs and Spices**

Although fruits and veggies are the stars of the Pesco-Mediterranean diet, herbs and spices deserve to be on your plate too. These plants are incredibly healthy and they will boost the nutritional value of your dishes too. By choosing the right herbs and spices, you can immediately jazz up your recipes to make your diet more interesting. You can even start your own herb garden at home to make sure that you always have something flavorful to add to your meals!

- **Legumes, Nuts, and Seeds**

Legumes are an excellent source of lean protein which makes them perfect for your diet. These tiny powerhouses are also chock-full of essential vitamins and minerals. As for nuts and seeds, they also provide you with proteins along with monounsaturated and polyunsaturated plant oils too. Instead of snacking on unhealthy processed snacks, why don't you satisfy your hunger with a handful of healthy nuts or seeds? Here are some examples of these foods to include in your diet:

o        Legumes and legume products like peanuts, pinto beans, kidney beans, tofu, lentils, peas, and hummus

o        Nuts like almonds, macadamias, walnuts, and hazelnuts.

o        Seeds like chia, hemp, and flaxseeds

o        Nut butters and seed butters

- **Whole Grains**

Whole grains like brown rice, quinoa, oats, and more are an excellent side dish for fish, seafood, and plant dishes too. They provide you with protein, fiber, and other essential nutrients. They also contain fewer additives and sugars compared to refined grains. Include whole grains, whole grains products, and pseudo-grains in your diet to make your meals more nutritious and filling.

These are the foods that you should focus on while following the Pesco-Mediterranean diet. While the number of food groups might seem very few, the food items within these groups will already provide you with an endless number of options for your daily meals and snacks. Aside from these, you may also consume the following in moderation while following the ideal diet:

- **Dairy Products**

Generally, you may have dairy products on this diet but in smaller amounts. Also, you want to focus on natural dairy products rather than the ones that are highly processed since this diet is all about whole foods. When it comes to dairy, the best options are plain yogurt, Greek yogurt, milk, and cheese. But if you opt to eliminate dairy from your diet, that would be okay too.

- **Eggs**

Eggs are very healthy as they contain vitamin D, protein, choline (to help with liver function and metabolism), and other healthy nutrients. Eating eggs once in a while or adding them to dishes is allowed on this diet, which means that if you love eggs, you don't have to give them up completely.

If you plan to eliminate dairy and eggs from your diet completely (even if you don't have to), you may have to monitor your calcium intake. Since these are the best sources of calcium, you should consult with your doctor and ask if you need to take calcium supplements along with your new diet.

For beverages, the preferred options are plain tea or coffee and water. While following this diet, especially during the transition period, you should make sure to keep yourself hydrated by drinking a lot of water. You may also have red wine in moderation along with your meals. By following this guide of foods to eat on the Pesco-Mediterranean diet, you will be able to enjoy a winning combination of foods that provide all of the fiber, vitamins, minerals, healthy fats, and phytochemicals your body needs to grow strong and healthy.

## What to Avoid

The Pesco-Mediterranean diet is neither strict nor restrictive but it does come with its own list of foods that you should minimize or avoid. But as you should already know by now, these are just recommendations on the diet. At the end of the day, your goal should be to learn how to clean up your diet by focusing on the list of foods in the previous section. While doing this, you should also try reducing your intake of the following foods:

- **Poultry, Meat, and Game**

Even if you choose to consume eggs and dairy products (which are derived from animals) or not, you should try to limit your intake of poultry, meat, or game. Although these foods contain nutrients, especially the organic and grass-fed varieties, they also contain high levels of saturated fats and cholesterol. These are counterproductive to your health goals, especially when you eat a lot of these foods. Some examples of these foods to avoid are:

- o        Red meat like beef, pork, lamb, or goat.
- o        Poultry like chicken, turkey, quail, or duck.
- o        Wild game like venison, goat, pheasant, or wild duck.

- **Processed Food Products**

Convenient and tasty as they are, processed foods aren't part of a healthy eating pattern like the Pesco-Mediterranean diet. These food products typically contain preservatives, additives, chemicals, and other unhealthy ingredients that can affect your body negatively. Therefore, if you want to lose weight, improve all aspects of your health, and enjoy other benefits, you should avoid processed food products as much as possible. Some examples of these foods to avoid are:

- o        Foods that contain artificial and added sugars like pastries, sodas, or candies.
- o        Processed meats like deli meats, hot dogs, or bacon.
- o        Ready-made pizza dough made with white flour.
- o        Refined grains like white pasta or white bread.

o           Refined oils like vegetable oil, corn oil, soybean oil, or hydrogenated oils.

o           Any food that is either processed or packaged, especially those which contain ingredients that sound too complex or difficult to read.

And that's about it!

As you can see, the Pesco-Mediterranean diet is truly simple and uncomplicated. You don't even have to make huge changes to your diet unless you only eat red meat, poultry, and processed foods. Even if you follow such a diet, you need to make healthier changes right now for the sake of your long-term health. Next up, you will learn how to start doing this...

## Basic Tips for Starting on the Diet

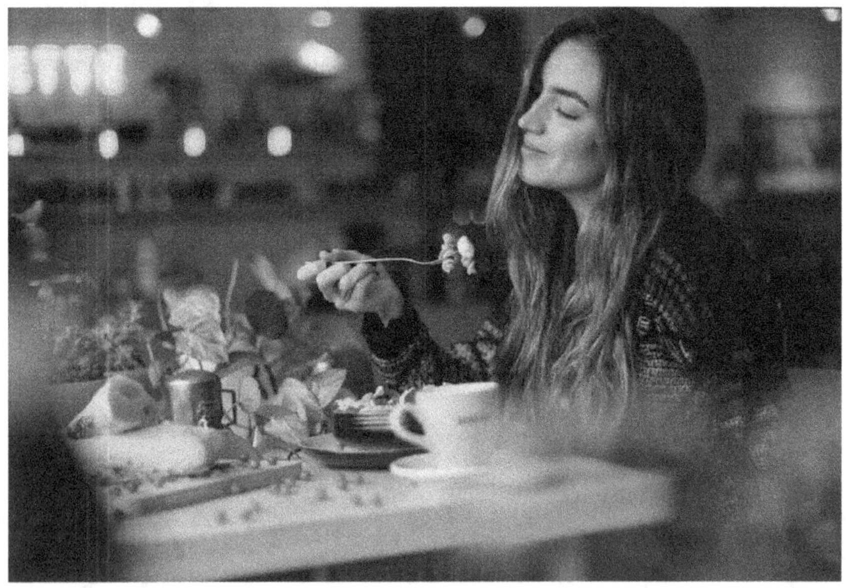

Now that you know what foods to eat and what to avoid, it's time to make a plan for how to start following the Pesco-Mediterranean diet. Since the food lists aren't that complex, creating this plan is very easy. To wrap up this chapter, let's go through some easy, practical, and effective tips to help you transition into this ideal diet for your health:

- **Stock up your pantry**

  First things first: you must clean up your pantry. For instance, if you have a lot of processed foods in your kitchen, it's time to get rid of these. You don't have to throw them away. Instead, you can pack everything in a box and donate the food so it doesn't go to waste. After that, you can start stocking up your pantry with whole, healthy foods that fit into your new diet.

- **Cook your meals**

  One of the most effective ways for you to stick with the Pesco-Mediterranean diet is by cooking your own meals. Although eating out or buying food is a lot easier and more convenient, doing this can also increase the likelihood of going back to your old eating habits. But if you learn how to cook your own meals, you can choose the dishes you will eat at every meal and the ingredients you will use to make these dishes.

  When it comes to cooking on the Pesco-Mediterranean diet, you may want to focus on healthy cooking methods like broiling, grilling, sautéing, roasting, baking, or even steaming your food. These methods are perfect for your new diet since the ingredients you will use can create amazingly healthy and flavorful dishes. Even if you have never tried cooking your own meals before, you can learn this skill easily. Start by looking for simple recipes online. You can also buy cookbooks that are specifically for the Pesco-Mediterranean diet. Either source will provide you with a wide range of dishes to keep you busy from simple recipes that take very little time to make to more complex recipes that require a lot of time and preparation.

- **Create a meal plan**

In line with the last point, you may want to consider meal planning too. If you don't want to cook because you have a job and you don't have time, meal planning can be a great help to you. Meal planning involves creating a plan for all of the meals you will eat within a given time frame—usually one week—then making all of these meals in a day.

Usually, you would set a day to plan your meals and buy the ingredients you need. Then you would set another day to cook all of those meals. Then all you have to do is store the meals you have prepared in the refrigerator and reheat those meals each day. Meal planning may take some getting used to. But once you get the hang of it, you will see how beneficial this process is.

- **Eat food that will make you healthy**

Right now, you might think that transitioning to a new diet is difficult and overwhelming, but it doesn't have to be. Since you already know which foods to eat and which ones to avoid, you can start creating a plan for yourself. To remind you, here's a rundown of the foods to focus on:

- Fruits and veggies—between 7 to 10 servings each day.
- Fish and seafood—start by having at least 2 servings each week.

o       Healthy fats and oils for cooking, making sauces or dressings, and to make your food more flavorful.

o       Whole grains and whole-grain products instead of refined grains.

o       Herbs and spices to make your dishes tastier and more interesting.

o       Moderate amounts of eggs and dairy products.

Whenever you are faced with food choices, always try to choose natural, whole, healthy foods that are suitable for the Pesco-Mediterranean diet. As time goes by, choosing such foods will come more naturally to you. This is when you know that you have successfully transitioned into the Pesco-Mediterranean diet.

- **Make sure you're well-hydrated**

Although the diet is already very healthy and nutrient-dense, you shouldn't forget to drink water. Water should be your go-to beverage all day, every day. Water helps with your digestion, it detoxifies your body, it makes you feel refreshed, and it offers cleansing benefits too. You can even add mint or fresh fruits to your water for a more interesting flavor.

- **Modify the diet as needed**

One of the best things about the Pesco-Mediterranean diet is its flexibility. You can plan your own meals, come up with your own strategies for how to follow the diet, and even make changes to your plans as the days go by. Even if you suffer from a medical condition and you need to follow a specialized diet, you can consult with your doctor about it. Together, you can come up with a plan for a Pesco-Mediterranean diet that will help improve the treatment for your condition.

- **Make your journey fun by focusing on positivity**

If you can start your Pesco-Mediterranean diet journey with positivity, your chance of succeeding will increase dramatically. Try not to think of it as a diet. Instead, you can consider this as a learning journey that will improve your overall lifestyle and health. As you make changes to your diet, try to enjoy your meals. Savor the flavors and if you choose to cook your own meals (which you should!), try to experiment with different ingredients and dishes. By doing this, you will make your journey much easier.

If you're considering the Pesco-Mediterranean diet, you should start as soon as you finish reading this book! If you aren't certain yet, you can give this diet a try for at least two weeks to see how it makes you feel. I promise you, after two weeks, you will already start feeling better. If you're not sure how to create a meal plan, you can research online or speak with a registered dietitian about it. The bottom line is, the Pesco-Mediterranean diet is simple and you can customize it to fit your own lifestyle.

Chapter 4:

# Focusing on Fiber

As you try to search for the best diet, you would have probably read or heard advice like, "Eat more fiber." This is because fiber is an essential nutrient that your body needs to stay healthy and function well.

Dietary fiber comes from the food you eat and its most important benefit is to aid in the relief or prevention of constipation. But this is not the only benefit that dietary fiber has to offer. Dietary fiber comes from the parts of the plants that you eat, specifically from the parts that your body cannot absorb or digest. Since it isn't digested like proteins, fats, or carbs, fiber simply passes through your digestive system without being broken down. There are two types of dietary fiber you can consume:

- **Insoluble fiber**

  Insoluble fiber helps move waste material through your whole digestive system while increasing the bulk of your stool in the process. This type of fiber is beneficial if you have irregular bowel movements or if you suffer from constipation. Some great sources of insoluble fiber are beans, nuts, veggies, and whole-wheat flour.

- **Soluble fiber**

  Soluble fiber forms a material with a gel-like texture after dissolving in water. This type of fiber helps lower your glucose and blood cholesterol levels making it essential too. Some great sources of soluble fiber are peas, apples, carrots, and oats.

The amount of fiber—both insoluble and soluble—in plant foods varies. Therefore, you should consume different kinds of high-fiber foods to make sure that you get all of the fiber you need each day. One of the most important reasons why plant foods are recommended on the Pesco-Mediterranean diet (and all other plant-based diets) is that they contain fiber. This nutrient offers a lot of health benefits, which we will discuss in the next section. But before that, let's go through some tips for how you can add more fiber to your diet:

- Find out which foods contain high amounts of fiber (we will discuss these too).
- Start your day with a high-fiber meal to jump-start your digestive system. For instance, you can have a bowl of bran or whole-grain cereal, which is filling and rich in fiber.
- Add more fruits and veggies to your diet. These contain fiber along with other essential nutrients you need to stay healthy.
- Consume a lot of legumes like lentils, peas, and beans. Add these legumes to various dishes to make them more nutritious while giving your meals a much-needed fiber boost.
- Opt for whole grains instead of refined grains. Whole grains like barley, bulgur wheat, wild rice, and brown rice are rich in dietary fiber. These will also keep you full for a longer time, which may help reduce your cravings too.
- Have high-fiber snacks too. Once in a while, snack on fiber-rich foods like raw veggies, fresh fruits, whole-grain pastries or crackers, nuts, seeds, or homemade popcorn. That way, your snacks will also help you consume your recommended daily fiber intake.

Adding more fiber into your diet doesn't have to be a difficult thing. As long as you make smarter food choices, this part of the Pesco-Mediterranean diet will already go a long way into improving your overall health in the long-run.

# The Many Benefits of Fiber

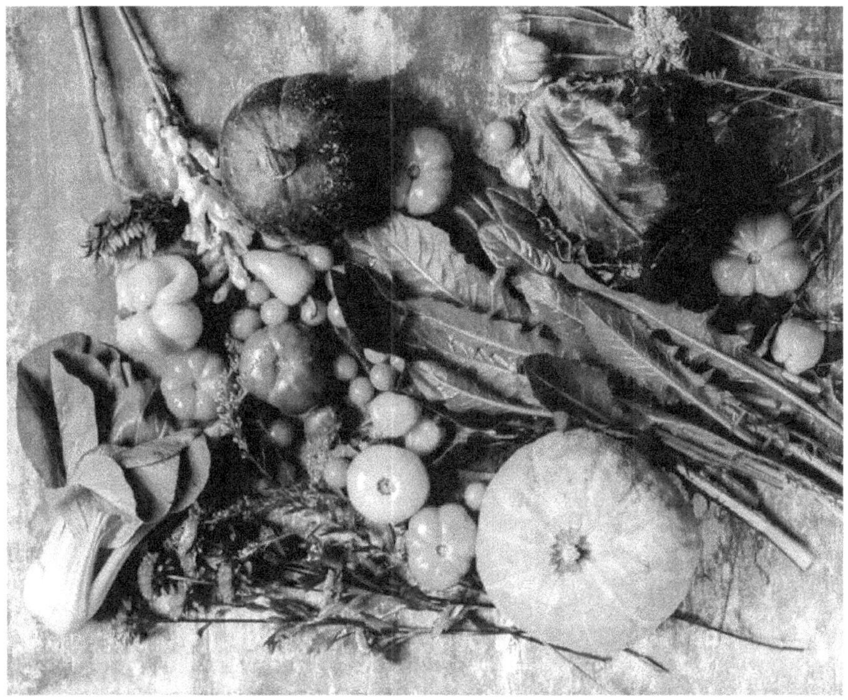

So we have already defined what fiber is, how you can add more fiber to your diet, and the fact that it is important to your health. The next question you may have right now is, 'Why?' With all of the vitamins, minerals, and nutrients different types of food have to offer, what makes fiber different? Before we go through the best fiber sources to add to your diet, let's discuss the wonderful health benefits this nutrient has to offer:

- **Improves your gut health**

    Your gut health or the health of your microbiome is extremely important. The microbiome contains bacteria and other microbes that live in your intestines and it is considered an "accessory organ." The function of the bacteria is to maintain the health of your intestines, regulate your immunity, improve your insulin sensitivity, affect the functioning of your nervous system, and even combat cancer.

When you take care of your gut, it will also take care of you. To keep your gut healthy, one of the best things you can feed it is fiber. The most beneficial foods for your microbiome are resistant starches and fermentable fibers. Since our cells don't possess the enzymes that can digest all fibers, this nutrient reaches your intestines without being broken down. Once there, the bacteria in your intestines are able to digest these fibers and start feeding on them. This, in turn, promotes the growth of your 'good' bacteria to improve your overall health. In fact, after just a few days of eating high-fiber foods, you will already notice good changes in how you feel.

- **Naturally detoxifies your body**

If you have been researching health and diets, you might have already read about juice cleanses. Popular as these are, especially for detoxification, you won't have to go on a juice cleanse (which I heard are quite challenging) if you consume enough fiber in your diet. Fiber helps detoxify your body by helping with the elimination of toxins from your GI tract.

In particular, soluble fiber absorbs compounds like unhealthy fats and excess estrogen, which can cause harm to the body. This effect prevents your body from absorbing the compounds. Insoluble fiber, on the other hand, makes your digestive system work more effectively by moving things along faster. This means that pesticides, mercury, and other potentially harmful substances in your food won't stay in your body for a long time. So if you want to detoxify your system regularly, focus on fiber.

- **Improves your bowel health**

Another benefit of fiber is that it helps make you more regular in terms of your bowel movements. Dietary fiber helps increase the size and weight of your stool while making it softer. A stool that is soft yet bulky passes through your system easily, which means that you won't end up suffering from constipation. If you usually pass stool that's too watery and loose, fiber can also be beneficial for you as it will absorb the water to make your stool bulkier and more solid.

- **Helps control your blood sugar levels**

For this, soluble fiber is more beneficial. By consuming foods that are rich in soluble fiber, your body's sugar absorption slows down, and this improves your blood sugar levels. Also, foods that are high in fiber are lower on the glycemic index, which helps reduce the likelihood of your blood sugar levels going too high. Of course, if you really want to enjoy this benefit, you may want to reduce your carb intake too, especially refined carbs.

- **Lowers your cholesterol levels**

Here's another benefit you can get from soluble fiber. By consuming foods rich in this type of fiber, your body's low-density lipoprotein cholesterol levels will go down. Since this is the "bad" type of cholesterol, this is a good thing. Fiber can also help reduce inflammation along with your blood pressure levels.

- **Reduced risk of type 2 diabetes and heart disease**

This is one of the greatest benefits of fiber. Several studies have consistently shown that an increased intake of fiber can help lower your risk of developing type 2 diabetes. This benefit comes from two other benefits fiber does to your body—stabilizing your blood sugar levels and helping you lose and maintain a healthy weight. These two benefits are significant factors that can help you avoid this chronic condition.

The more fiber you eat, the more you reduce your risk of heart disease as well. One of the reasons this happens is that fiber tends to absorb excess cholesterol in your body.

- **Helps you lose weight**

Since high-fiber foods are more filling, you will feel full and satisfied for a longer period of time. This means that there is a lower likelihood of craving for snacks frequently throughout the day because you won't feel hungry right away. This benefit combined with the fact that high-fiber foods generally contain fewer calories will help you lose weight. This is especially true for foods that contain soluble fiber.

By increasing your fiber intake, you will notice yourself shedding those stubborn excess pounds. Once you have reached a healthy weight, you can maintain this by continuing with your high-fiber diet. That way, you can stay healthy in the long-run and avoid the development of various chronic diseases that are associated with being overweight or obese.

- **Reduces your risk of cancer**

Although an increase in fiber can combat cancer, this is most applicable to colorectal cancer, which is the type of cancer that typically leads to death. All foods that are high in fiber also contain a wide range of antioxidants and nutrients that contribute to this benefit too. Since fiber keeps your gut and the rest of your digestive system healthy, it also helps you avoid this devastating condition. Some studies have even suggested that fiber can also help combat breast cancer. Although more studies are needed for this benefit, it's still something to look forward to.

- **Helps you live a longer life**

With all of the benefits fiber has to offer, it's only natural that you will lead a longer life. By increasing your fiber intake, your body will undergo a lot of positive changes, which will help you avoid chronic conditions. This means that you will be healthier and this will add more years to your life.

Now you know how important fiber is to your diet. To enjoy all of these benefits, you have to know which foods to focus on—and that is what we will discuss next.

# The Best Fiber Sources to Focus On

As you can see, fiber is very important. However, not all types of food contain fiber. If you want to add more fiber to your diet, you can do this by adding certain foods to your meals or snacks. The Pesco-Mediterranean diet is high in fiber, which is one of the reasons why it's so beneficial. If you have been following the Standard American diet all your life, chances are, you wouldn't have consumed the daily recommended intake of this nutrient. But if you make the switch to the Pesco-Mediterranean diet, you will start noticing improvements in your health that typically come with a high-fiber diet. If you're wondering which foods are high in fiber, here are some of the best options:

- **Almonds**

These are a very common type of tree nut that can be eaten on their own or used in sweet and savory dishes. Apart from fiber, almonds are also high in vitamin E, magnesium, manganese, healthy fats, and other healthy nutrients. Add almonds to various recipes or have a handful of them as a snack to give yourself a fiber boost.

- **Apples**

These fruits are tasty, satisfying, and there are so many varieties to try that you will never get bored. Apples are nutrient-rich and they contain a good amount of fiber too.

- **Artichokes**

Although this veggie isn't as popular as others, it is one of the best sources of fiber. Since artichokes also contain a wide range of nutrients, they really belong in your diet.

- **Avocados**

Most healthy diets recommend adding avocado because this is one of the healthiest fruits out there. Avocados are loaded with vitamin C, vitamin E, magnesium potassium, healthy fats, B-vitamins, and fiber. The best part is, avocados are extremely versatile, which means that you can eat them in different ways.

- **Bananas**

Bananas are high in vitamin B6, potassium, vitamin C, and fiber. Unripe bananas also contain resistant starch, which is a type of carb that works like fiber since it isn't digestible.

- **Beets**

This is a type of root vegetable that contains various essential nutrients aside from fiber. Beets also contain inorganic nitrates, which can help improve your body's regulation of blood sugar and your performance while working out.

- **Broccoli**

This belongs to the family of cruciferous veggies and it's one of the most nutrient-dense veggies out there. Broccoli is loaded with vitamins, minerals, antioxidants, and powerful nutrients that combat cancer. Aside from being high in fiber, this veggie also contains more protein compared to other veggies. Whether raw or cooked, broccoli is an excellent choice.

- **Brussels sprouts**

This is another type of cruciferous veggie although this one isn't as popular as broccoli. Brussels sprouts are rich in folate, potassium, vitamin K, fiber, and powerful antioxidants. Add them to your veggie recipes to make your meals healthier.

- **Carrots**

This root vegetable is crunchy, tasty, and very nutritious. It contains beta carotene, a powerful antioxidant that your body transforms into vitamin A. This high-fiber veggie also contains magnesium, vitamin B6, vitamin K, and other beneficial nutrients.

- **Chia seeds**

These seeds are now considered superfoods and have become a huge trend all over the world. They are extremely nutritious, high in fiber, and contain other essential nutrients like calcium, phosphorus, and magnesium.

- **Chickpeas**

This is a type of legume that's chock-full of nutrients, minerals, protein, and fiber. If you like hummus, then you will like chickpeas because these form the base of the popular dip. You can also roast chickpeas for a healthy and tasty snack.

- **Dark chocolate**

Being one of the tastiest foods in the world, you should be happy to know that dark chocolate is high in fiber. Surprisingly, this bittersweet treat is also high in nutrients and antioxidants. When it comes to dark chocolate, choose varieties that have a minimum of 70% cocoa without added sugar.

- **Edamame**

These are immature soybeans and they have a lovely texture and taste. Edamame is an excellent plant-based source of amino acids and fiber. You can find edamame in pods or already shelled.

- **Kidney beans**

These legumes are loaded with nutrients, plant-based proteins, and fiber. Add them to stews, soups, and other recipes to make them more savory, filling, and satisfying.

- **Lentils**

Aside from being extremely economical, lentils are also high in fiber and important nutrients. Lentils are very versatile too so it's easy to make them part of your diet.

- **Oats**

These are some of the healthiest grains in the world. They're fiber-rich and they also contain antioxidants, vitamins, and minerals. Oats contain glucan, a potent soluble fiber that can be very beneficial to your cholesterol and blood sugar levels.

- **Pears**

This yummy fruit is sweet, crunchy, and very healthy. It's another high-fiber fruit that you can enjoy as a snack or even use in various desserts.

- **Popcorn**

Snacking on popcorn can increase your fiber intake. As long as you make your own popcorn instead of opting for microwavable popcorn products, you can enjoy this low-calorie treat to help increase your fiber intake. Of course, it's best to avoid high-calorie toppings like caramel, butter, or flavored powders.

- **Quinoa**

Just like chia seeds, this pseudo-cereal is considered one of the most powerful superfoods on the planet. Because of this, it has become a huge trend among health enthusiasts and those who are interested in starting a new diet. This fiber-rich grain is loaded with protein, zinc, potassium, antioxidants, and other nutrients to improve your health.

- **Raspberries**

These berries might be small but they have a very potent flavor. They contain vitamin C, manganese, and fiber along with other healthy vitamins and minerals. Snack on these healthy berries on their own or add them to sweet dishes.

- **Split peas**

These are made from seeds of peas that have been peeled, split, and dried. The most popular way to use these is in split pea soup. Of course, you can use split peas in other recipes too.

- **Strawberries**

If you can get your hands on fresh strawberries, you can add more fiber to your day while enjoying the lovely taste of this fruit. Strawberries are rich in nutrients like manganese, vitamin C, and a wide range of potent antioxidants.

- **Sweet potatoes**

This tuber has a wonderful sweet flavor and it's very filling. Like carrots, sweet potatoes are rich in beta carotene. They also contain fiber, B-vitamins, and different minerals. Use these in sweet and savory dishes for a nutritious fiber boost.

- ## Other high-fiber foods

Apart from these foods, here are other options that contain good amounts of fiber:

- o        Baked beans
- o        Barley
- o        Black beans (cooked)
- o        Blackberries
- o        Blueberries
- o        Brown rice
- o        Coconut
- o        Kale
- o        Lima beans (cooked)
- o        Pecans
- o        Pistachios
- o        Pumpkin seeds
- o        Spinach
- o        Sunflower seeds
- o        Tomatoes
- o        Walnuts
- o        Whole grains

When it comes to fiber, it's best to get this nutrient from whole foods. When you start following the Pesco-Mediterranean diet, you will be able to get enough fiber each day. But if you think that you aren't getting enough fiber, you can ask your doctor if you need to take fiber supplements. You may need this, especially while you are transitioning into the Pesco-Mediterranean diet. But when your body has already adjusted to the unique eating pattern, you might not have to take these fiber supplements.

Chapter 5:

# Legumes and Whole Grains as

# Nutritional Powerhouses

Legumes and grains are usually paired with each other in various recipes and meals. Some common combinations are rice and red beans, corn chips with bean dip, and black bean casserole with quinoa, for example. The main reason for this is that legumes and grains work well together to create healthy, filling dishes that have wonderful flavors and textures.

Whole grains are grains that are still intact or which still possess all the layers of the grain. Whole grains contain various nutrients and active substances that help prevent diseases while providing adequate nourishment to the body. When grains are processed, this tends to remove several nutrients. This is why whole grains are considered healthier compared to refined grains. Legumes, on the other hand, are the seeds or fruits of plants from a specific family. These nutritious foods are an important part of plant-rich diets as they contain various vitamins, minerals, and nutrients. Many studies have shown how beneficial legumes can be. One such study showed that the increase in the consumption of legumes, whole grains, and other plant sources helps lower the risk of type 2 diabetes, stroke, high blood pressure, and heart disease (Polak, R., et. al., 2015).

People all over the world pair legumes and whole grains as part of their regular diets. These combinations can be sweet or savory depending on the other ingredients included in the dishes. These pairings are especially common in Asian countries but they are also quite common in Greece and other countries in the Mediterranean region. Some examples of these dishes are:

- Congee, which is a type of thick porridge that is sometimes paired with red or mung beans with sugar. This is a common dish in China.
- In India, congee is also quite common, but it is prepared using other types of grains like millet.
- In Latin America, particularly in Brazil and Costa Rica, a traditional dish called "Gallo Pinto" is very common, which consists of beans and rice.
- There is a popular soup dish in that Italy consists of veggies, beans, and pasta is called "Pasta e Fagioli.'
- A dish known as "Gigandes Plaki" is a traditional appetizer in Greece. This consists of bread with a dipping sauce of tomato sauce with large white beans.
- In Africa, they have several dishes that combine beans and grains. One such example is bean stew served with bread made from teff grains called injera bread. This dish is popular in Ethiopia.

These are just some examples of classic legume and whole grain pairings that are both nutritious and delicious. If you try to search for more dishes online, you will discover a lot more!

Legumes and whole grains are cooked and prepared in different ways. This versatility makes them an excellent choice in the Pesco-Mediterranean diet because you can also pair these food groups with all the other food groups you are encouraged to focus on. By doing this, you will increase the likelihood of enjoying all the health benefits legumes and whole grains have to offer.

# The Benefits of Legumes and Whole Grains

On their own, legumes and whole grains have wonderful health benefits you can look forward to. When put together, these nutritious food groups provide you with incredibly healthy nutrients. If you're wondering why these tiny powerhouses are an essential part of the Pesco-Mediterranean diet, here are some benefits they have to offer:

- Beans and other legumes are very cheap and yet, they are rich sources of fiber, complex carbs, protein, and various micronutrients.

- Beans contain resistant starch and short-chain sugar polymers (oligosaccharides), which act as prebiotics. This means that they are beneficial for your GI tract.

- Beans also contain various antioxidants in the form of chemicals like phytic acid, saponins, and phenolic compounds. These provide protective effects on the body.

- Beans are low-sodium food that helps regulate blood sugar levels and suppresses appetite. They come in dried or canned varieties, which you would have to prepare in different ways before adding them to dishes.

- Since legumes are high in protein, they help with the regulation of various metabolic processes.

- Whole grains improve the overall quality of your diet to help reduce your risk of chronic diseases like type 2 diabetes and heart disease.

- Consuming a wide variety of whole grains can help reduce your diet's overall glycemic index too.

- Legumes and whole grains can help you lose weight and maintain a healthy weight.

- Legumes and whole grains are extremely versatile as you can use them in salads, appetizers, soups, stews, desserts, and both cold and hot entrées. They're readily available, nutrient-dense, and they have very adaptable flavor profiles.

- Combining legumes and whole grains provide you with all of the essential amino acids you need. Since legumes and grains are incomplete proteins, combining them in dishes allows them to complement each other and form complete proteins. This means that they are an excellent substitute for animal proteins.

With all of these benefits, you would think that legumes and whole grains are some of the most popular foods in the world. However, this isn't always the case, especially since many diets don't focus on whole grains and legumes. Some diets even discourage their consumption, especially low-carb diets. Now that you know how healthy these foods are, it's time to bring them back into your dishes. The good news is that the Pesco-Mediterranean diet encourages the consumption of legumes and whole grains. Now, all you have to do is find out which are the healthiest ones.

## Healthy and Tasty Legumes

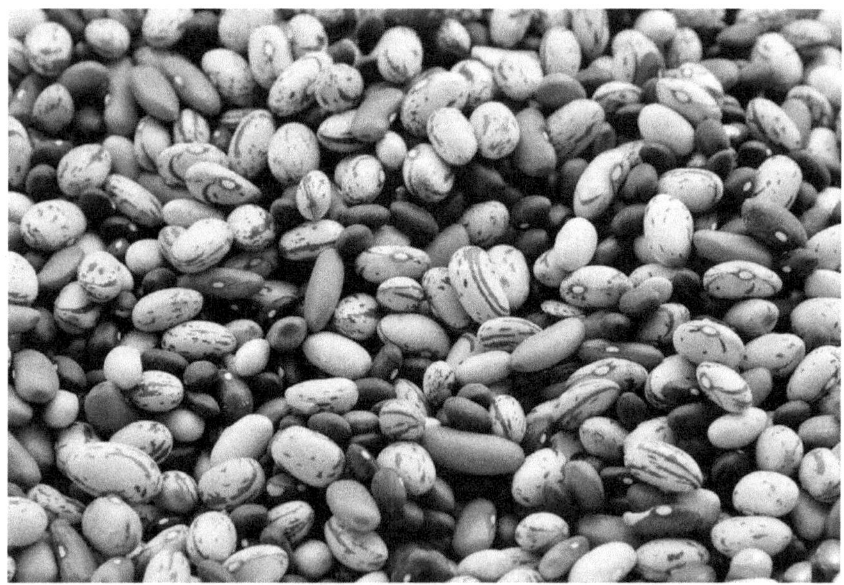

Legumes, which include beans, are the seeds of fruits of the Fabaceae plant family. Small as they are, legumes are rich in fiber, B vitamins, and other valuable nutrients. Since the Pesco-Mediterranean diet is more plant-based than animal-based, legumes can serve as an excellent replacement for meat. Legumes will provide you with plant-based protein too, which is why they are a wonderful addition to your diet. Here are the most nutritious legumes to eat:

- **Black beans**

These beans are an excellent source of fiber, folate, and protein. By consuming black beans, you don't have to worry about spikes in your blood sugar levels because they have a low glycemic index. These beans can also help reduce the risk of weight gain and diabetes.

- **Chickpeas**

Some people know these legumes as garbanzo beans and they contain a lot of protein and fiber. Adding chickpeas to your diet can help you lose weight while reducing your risk of heart disease and even cancer. Chickpeas are especially beneficial at improving your insulin sensitivity and reducing your blood sugar and cholesterol levels.

- **Kidney beans**

These are some of the most popular beans and usually, people enjoy these beans with rice. Kidney beans aid in the slow absorption of sugar, which leads to a reduction in your blood sugar levels. These versatile beans can also help reduce the risk factors of metabolic syndrome and diabetes thanks to all of the healthy nutrients they contain.

- **Lentils**

Another popular type of legumes, lentils are very common in plant-based diets. These legumes have similar benefits as chickpeas. They also help improve your bowel functions by improving your gut health. With all of these benefits and more, lentils are considered the healthiest legumes on the planet. They're easy to cook and they add nutrients to your dishes. You don't even have to soak them before cooking. Adding lentils to stews, soups, and other dishes will provide you with vegetarian proteins and other essential nutrients.

- **Navy beans**

Some people know navy beans as haricot beans and they are an excellent source of B-vitamins, minerals, and fiber. Because of their high-fiber content, these beans may help reduce the symptoms of metabolic syndrome. One reason for this is that navy beans help increase the levels of HDL or 'good' cholesterol in the body. These beans can also help you lose weight while improving your blood pressure and blood sugar levels.

- **Peanuts**

This may come as a surprise to a lot of people but peanuts aren't actually nuts—they're legumes. Aside from fiber, peanuts contain polyunsaturated fats, monounsaturated fats, B-vitamins, and protein. Some studies have suggested that adding peanuts to your diet may help reduce your risk of diabetes, stroke, heart disease, and even cancer. However, many people are allergic to peanuts. Therefore, you should make sure that you don't have a peanut allergy first before consuming this high-fiber legume.

- **Peas**

There are many types of peas for you to choose from and they all pack a lot of protein and fiber. Pea proteins and fibers are commonly used as supplements because they offer a lot of benefits. Some examples of these benefits are a reduction in insulin resistance and a reduction of belly fat. Eating peas can also make you feel full for a longer time. The fiber found in peas can also improve your gut health, which, as you already know, is essential for your overall health and well-being.

- **Pinto beans**

These beans are very common in Mexican dishes and you can have them fried, mashed, or whole. The main benefit of pinto beans is that they help lower your cholesterol levels. These beans help increase the levels of HDL cholesterol while decreasing the levels of LDL cholesterol. Pinto beans can also promote the production of a short-chain fatty acid known as propionate that is good for your gut health. These legumes are also high in essential minerals like potassium, iron, manganese, and phosphorus. They can even help you combat flu and colds by strengthening your immune system.

- **Soybeans**

These are very common legumes and they can come in different forms. Apart from fiber, soybeans are rich in isoflavones. This is a powerful antioxidant that offers a number of health benefits, one of which is a reduced risk of developing certain types of cancer like breast cancer and various gastrointestinal cancers. Just like other high-fiber legumes, soybeans can also help reduce the risk of heart disease while regulating your blood cholesterol and blood pressure levels.

While these legumes are considered the healthiest, other legumes belong in your diet too. After all, the Pesco-Mediterranean diet is all about healthy, whole foods. To make things more interesting, try to incorporate a variety of ingredients in your dishes. That way, you will always feel motivated to stick with your diet because you will never run out of delicious options.

## Healthy and Tasty Whole Grains

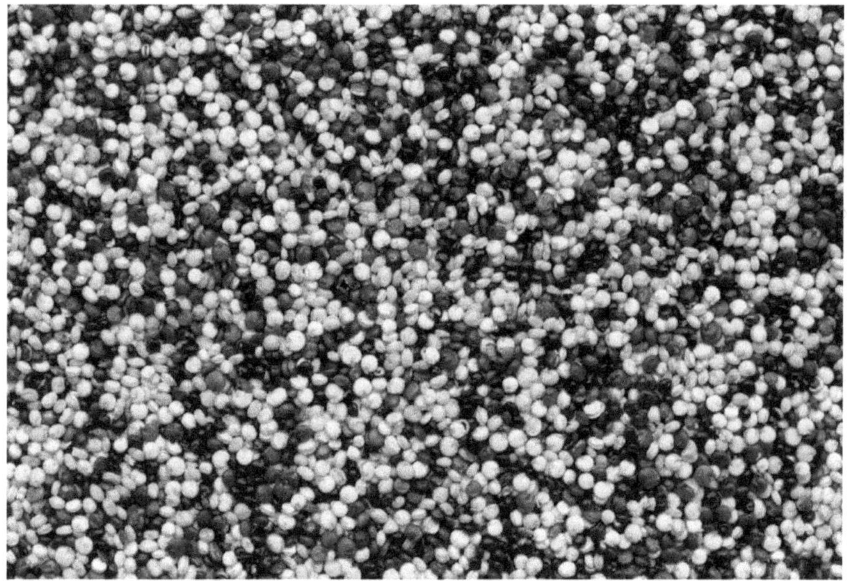

All over the world, grains are a very common staple in kitchens. Grains are composed of the nutrient-dense outer layer known as the bran, the nutrient-dense embryo known as the germ, and the food supply of the germ, which is the endosperm. For whole grains, all of these layers are intact, which makes them more nutrient-rich compared to refined grains. Now, let's go through some of the healthiest grains to include in your Pesco-Mediterranean diet:

- **Amaranth**

This is one of the ancient grains that are rich in essential vitamins and minerals. Although not very common, amaranth is actually very easy to cook and this grain provides a lovely texture to dishes. To give your meals a boost of nutrients, add this grain to stews, soups, or salads.

- **Barley**

This is one of the more underrated grains out there even though it's really healthy. You can enjoy whole-grain barley or cut and milled barley that comes in the form of steel-cut barley or barley grits. You can use these to make barley porridge. Barley contains a wide range of nutrients that offers health benefits like bone support, heart health, anti-inflammatory properties, blood pressure regulation, and promoting the health of your gut too. Barley also contains soluble fiber, which comes with its own range of benefits.

- **Brown rice**

Leaving the bran on rice gives you brown rice. This variety of rice is a great source of protein, vitamins, minerals, and dietary fiber. A cup of this rice also provides you with the mineral manganese that offers protective benefits against damage caused by free radicals.

- **Buckwheat**

This is a type of pseudo-cereal that's chock-full of B-vitamins, fiber, and different kinds of minerals. This gluten-free grain improves the health of your gut, promotes weight loss, and protects your heart.

- **Bulgur or cracked wheat**

This whole grain is so versatile that you can add it to salads, soups, and even stuff vegetables with it for a filling meal. Bulgur is a low-fat grain that is rich in fiber, iron, manganese, and magnesium. It has anti-inflammatory benefits, it promotes the health of your heart, and it can even help your body combat certain types of cancer. However, since bulgur contains gluten, you should avoid it if you have celiac disease or gluten intolerance.

- **Millet**

This is another grain that isn't as commonly consumed as it should be. Millet is naturally gluten-free and it offers an alkalizing effect. Although this grain isn't as protein-rich as other varieties, it does contain essential nutrients like magnesium, iron, and potassium. Another ancient grain, millet is amazingly nutritious, which means that it also offers amazing benefits to your health.

- **Oats**

If you want to start your day off right, why don't you enjoy a bowl of oats? Oats are high in fiber, which means that you will feel full after eating a bowl. And if you add fresh fruits to the mix, you will definitely be eating for your health. Oats contain beta-glucan, a type of fiber that will help lower your cholesterol levels. This healthy grain also contains B-vitamins, magnesium, selenium, and manganese.

- **Popcorn**

When it comes to snacks, popcorn is an excellent option. This whole-grain is low in calories but high in fiber, zinc, copper, magnesium, phosphorus, manganese, and B-vitamins. When it comes to popcorn, it's best to cook it yourself to avoid unhealthy ingredients that are typically added to popcorn snacks like caramel, butter, and a lot of salt.

- **Quinoa**

This is one of the most popular grains in the world and it's considered a 'superfood." Quinoa is rich in plant-protein and it also contains other essential nutrients like amino acids, fiber, calcium, iron, and B-vitamins. This is very versatile, which means that you can use it in a wide range of dishes.

- **Spelt**

This ancient whole wheat is nutritionally similar to modern varieties of whole wheat. The only difference is that it contains more protein and zinc. Spelt also contains phytic acid and other antinutrients that help reduce iron and zinc absorption from your gut. But you should know that spelt also contains gluten, which means that it's not suitable for everyone.

- **Teff**

This might be a very small grain but when it comes to nutrients, teff is a powerhouse. It's rich in magnesium, calcium, fiber, protein, and potassium. This is a gluten-free grain that's easy to cook. It also contains a wide range of minerals to make you healthier.

- **Wild rice**

The best nutrients this grain has to offer are zinc, vitamin B3, fiber, and protein. It also contains phytonutrients and antioxidants, which improve health. However, wild rice takes a longer time to cook compared to other grains.

- **Whole-grain rye**

This is another type of grain that contains gluten. If you don't have any problem with the consumption of gluten, you should definitely add this to your diet. Rye is incredibly high in dietary fiber and other essential nutrients. For this grain, you should opt for whole-grain rye since refined varieties typically contain fewer nutrients.

When it comes to whole grains, there are many options for you on the Pesco-Mediterranean diet. Mix things up and try different types of grains to make your diet healthier and more interesting.

# Chapter 6:

# Nutritious Fish and Seafood

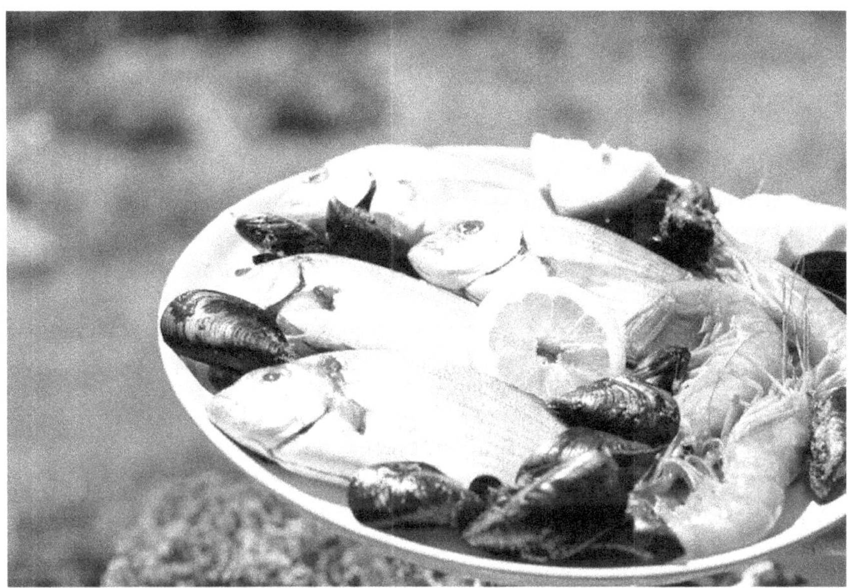

If you go to health professionals like dieticians and doctors to ask how you can improve your health, they will probably recommend that you add more fish to your diet. Healthy diets include eating fish at least twice a week. Since you will be relying on fish and seafood as your main animal protein source on the Pesco-Mediterranean diet, you can increase this number.

Fish is one of the healthiest groups of foods in the world. Most types of fish are rich in vitamin D, protein, omega-3 fatty acids, and other essential nutrients. These nutrients will boost the health of your brain, your body, and improve your overall well-being. Seafood is an important group of food too. It includes sea vegetables, shellfish, and even fish. There are different types of seafood that you can eat, most of which are extremely nutrient-dense. Aside from being rich in omega-3s, seafood is also high in protein while being low in fat and calories. Because of this, both fish and seafood make the perfect sources of animal protein on the Pesco-Mediterranean diet. In fact, several studies have shown that consuming fish and seafood can help decrease the risk of chronic diseases like stroke, hypertension, and heart attack.

Although fish and seafood are highly recommended, some people don't feel comfortable consuming these foods because of the belief that they are high in cholesterol. Although these foods do contain cholesterol, the type of cholesterol in fish and seafood doesn't get transferred to the blood directly. If you really want to keep your cholesterol levels in check, you should avoid foods that are high in trans and saturated fats. These are the ones that go directly to your blood and cause a number of adverse side effects.

Another common concern that is associated with the consumption of fish and seafood is mercury content. When consumed in excess, this chemical element can cause nerve and brain damage. The good news is that fish and seafood varieties that contain the highest omega-3 fatty acids also happen to be the ones that have the lowest mercury content. Later, we will go through the healthiest fish and seafood varieties to focus on while following the Pesco-Mediterranean diet. But before that, let's see how these foods can be beneficial to your health.

## Why Do You Need to Add Fish and Seafood to Your Plate?

Fish and seafood are highly beneficial, which is why they are the stars of the Pesco-Mediterranean diet when it comes to animal protein. As you plan your transition into this healthy diet, you should include a variety of these healthy foods in your dishes. By doing this, you will enjoy the following benefits:

## *Fish*

There are so many different types of fish you can choose from and all of them contain essential nutrients to help you become healthy and strong. Here are some of the most important benefits fish has to offer:

- **Contain crucial nutrients for development**

    This benefit mainly comes from the high omega-3 fatty acid content of fish. Omega-3 fatty acids are essential for development, which is why fish is recommended for women who are either pregnant or breastfeeding. If you belong to these categories (or even if you don't), opt for low-mercury fish to ensure that you are only getting the beneficial compounds without the risk of negative side effects.

- **High in essential nutrients**

    Fish is high in essential nutrients that are typically lacking in Western diets. These nutrients include iodine, high-quality protein, iron, zinc, and other vitamins and minerals. Fatty fish are especially important as these contain the highest concentration of these essential minerals. Since fish is an important part of the Pesco-Mediterranean diet, this means that you will always be consuming these nutrients whenever you eat fish.

- **Excellent dietary source of vitamin D**

    Vitamin D is one of the rarest vitamins you can get from food, which is why most people are either low or deficient in this vitamin. Fortunately, fish is one of the best sources of dietary vitamin D on the planet. This is especially true for herring, salmon, and other types of fatty fish.


- **Promotes your overall health**


With all of the nutrients fish contains, it's only natural that eating this food will promote your overall health. Here are some examples of the good things that can happen within your body as part of your health improvement:


  - The health of your brain will improve, which means that the age-related decline of your mental health will slow down too.
  - The omega-3 fatty acid content helps improve eye health while reducing the risk of age-related macular degeneration. The nutrients in fish can even help improve your night vision.
  - Consuming fish is also beneficial for your joints. This is another benefit that comes from the omega-3 fatty acid content of fish.
  - You may notice that the natural glow of your skin is coming back as the vitamin content in fish helps preserve your skin's moisture.
  - Fish helps improve your body's immune function thanks to its high antioxidant content.
  - The vitamin D content of fish helps improve the quality of your sleep. This is an important benefit as getting enough sleep also improves other aspects of your health.


- **Offers protective benefits**

Apart from improving your health, the consumption of fish can also offer a number of protective benefits. This means that following the Pesco-Mediterranean diet, which includes a lot of fish can offer the following advantages:

- o       Lowers your risk of strokes and heart attacks since fish is one of the best heart-healthy foods out there.
- o       Reduces your risk of developing autoimmune diseases like type-1 diabetes and multiple sclerosis. This is mainly due to the high vitamin D and omega-3 fatty acid content.
- o       It may help treat or prevent depression. Since this is a type of mental condition and fish helps improve the health of your brain, this is one benefit you can potentially look forward to.
- o       It can also help prevent asthma, especially in children. Although this benefit doesn't seem to be evident in adults.

## *Seafood*

Aside from fish, you can also consume other types of seafood on the Pesco-Mediterranean diet. Seafood like shrimps, crab, lobster, and others are an excellent source of animal protein, which makes them ideal for this healthy plant-rich diet. Seafood shares the same benefits as fish but you can also enjoy other benefits such as:

- •    **Contain healthy fats**

Generally, seafood contains minimal amounts of total and saturated fats. Most types of shellfish and fish contain 5% of fat while fatty fish like salmon and mackerel only contain up to

15% of fat. The good news is, most of this fat is considered healthy fat like omega-3s and polyunsaturated fats, which are beneficial to your health. Also, seafood contains minimal amounts of cholesterol so you don't have to worry about your cholesterol levels getting elevated by eating dishes that contain seafood.

- **High in protein but low in calories**

Another benefit of seafood is that it's low in calories. Since fish and seafood will be your main protein source, weight loss is a natural effect of this diet. Also, the protein content of seafood is easier for your body to digest, which means that your body will be able to absorb it more easily compared to protein from poultry and red meat.

- **Rich in essential vitamins and minerals**

Aside from vitamin D and omega-3s, seafood also offers a wide range of essential vitamins and minerals such as B-complex vitamins, vitamin A, selenium, zinc, and more. All of these provide beneficial effects like healthier skin, healthier vision, and healthy bone development. These nutrients also improve the functions of your immune system and thyroid gland. They also promote the efficiency of red blood cell production while protecting your body against cell damage.

For both fish and seafood, another wonderful benefit is that they are easy to cook. If you try to search for fish and seafood recipes online, you will discover endless options. As you will soon experience (once you start cooking Pesco-Mediterranean-friendly fish and seafood recipes), all of these dishes are scrumptious and satisfying. And for the final benefit, fish and seafood offer plenty of choices for you to choose from. Combine these options with all the other foods you can eat on the Pesco-Mediterranean diet and you will never get bored. This is why the diet is considered highly sustainable and enjoyable too.

## The Most Nutrient-Dense Fish

Most types of fish are rich in essential nutrients, B-vitamins, and protein. But just like all other foods, there are some types of fish that are much healthier, and generally better for you. Although all fish are ideal for the Pesco-Mediterranean diet, you may want to increase your intake of the following fish:

- **Albacore Tuna**

  For this tuna, you can enjoy the canned version because it's so versatile and convenient. Of course, if you can get your hands on fresh Albacore tuna, even better! This fish is rich in omega-3 fatty acids, as well as protein. Use this fish in various dishes for a boost of flavor and nutrients.

- **Anchovies**

  These fish might be small but they pack a huge punch in terms of nutrition. Anchovies are small, oily fish that have a strong flavor. Often, they are either salt-cured or preserved in brine. It's more common to use anchovies in dishes instead of eating them on their own. Either way, they contain a lot of vitamins, omega-3s, and nutrients to boost your health.

- **Arctic char**

  This fish belongs to the salmon family and its flavor and nutrient profile are similar to salmon too. It has firm meat that becomes flaky when cooked, and it's rich in healthy fats. The flesh of this fish ranges from pale pink to dark red.

- **Cod**

This white fish has flaky flesh and it's very common in Mediterranean dishes. It's rich in niacin, vitamin B12, and phosphorus. If you're not used to eating fish, you can start with this one as it has a mild flavor and a lovely texture. Apart from being high in protein, cod is also free of saturated fat.

- **Fish roe**

Although not technically fish, this is still a healthy option as it comes from fish. These are fish eggs and they are very nutritious. Fish roe contains vitamin D, protein, omega-3, and other nutrients. There are several types of fish roe and they have various colors, flavors, and textures.

- **Freshwater trout**

This fish is high in protein but low in calories. It's rich in B-vitamins and omega-3 fatty acids making it an amazing addition to your Pesco-Mediterranean diet. Freshwater trout also happens to be a great source of dietary iodine.

- **Freshwater whitefish**

This fish is related to salmon but its flesh is pure white when raw. It's rich in omega-3 fatty acids and healthy fats.

- **Halibut**

Halibut has a clean taste, a firm texture, and lots of protein. This is a very healthy type of fish as it also contains B-vitamins, vitamin D, phosphorus, and selenium.

- **Herring**

This is another fish that is rich in vitamin B-12 along with other vitamins. Since this is also an oily fish, it is chock-full of omega-3s too. You can prepare herring in different ways like smoking, drying, pickling, or salting. Among all of these, smoked herring seems to be the preferred option. Although this is a small fish, it has a strong flavor making it a wonderful addition to dishes.

- **Mackerel**

When it comes to healthy fish varieties, the best ones are oily fish. This is another variety of oily fish that contains the essential vitamins, minerals, and nutrients you need. However, fresh mackerel tends to spoil quickly so you must make sure to eat it right away, cure it, or refrigerate it.

- **Mahi-mahi**

This tropical fish has firm flesh and it can be cooked in different ways. It's tasty, healthy, and it fits right into the Pesco-Mediterranean diet.

- **Perch**

This is another type of whitefish with a medium texture. It has a mild taste and although not very common, it's quite versatile too. Just like other whitefish, perch is very nutritious.

- **Rainbow trout**

For this fish, the farmed variety is safer than the wild version because the former is protected against contaminants. This tasty fish is very healthy and it's also one of the best options if you're considering the environmental impact of your diet too.

- **Salmon**

When it comes to healthy fish, salmon is one of the best and most popular options. This oily fish has flesh that ranges from red to orange and it's an excellent source of essential nutrients like B-vitamins, omega-3 fatty acids, protein, and more. Although farmed salmon is the more economical option, wild salmon is much healthier. Either way, adding this dish to your diet will not only make it healthier, but it will add more variety to your diet.

- **Sardines**

Also one of the healthy oily fishes to add to your diet, sardines contain a lot of vitamins. Canned sardines are much more convenient and they are even considered more nutritious because you would consume the whole fish, bones, organs, and all. Sardines are affordable, nutritious, and they're an excellent source of vitamin D, among other nutrients.

- **Sprats**

This fish isn't very common but it belongs to a family of common fish like herring, sardines, and anchovies. Small as sprats are, they offer a lot of nutrients.

- **Striped bass**

This is one variety of bass which has a flaky but firm texture. Along with a full flavor, striped bass is rich in protein, omega-3s, vitamin B12, phosphorus, and manganese. Other common varieties of bass are sea bass and largemouth bass.

- **Swordfish**

This is one of the bigger fish you can add to your diet and it also happens to be a predator of the sea. It's high in omega-3 fatty acids although some people are concerned with its potentially high mercury content.

- **Tuna**

This saltwater fish is one of the most common in the world along with salmon. Canned tuna is very popular but you can also enjoy it fresh. This fish is rich in vitamin D, phosphorus, and protein. Whether canned or fresh, tuna is extremely versatile. You can make this the star of your dish or one of the ingredients for more complex dishes on your Pesco-Mediterranean diet.

- **Wild Alaskan pollock**

This wild-caught fish has a light texture and a mild flavor. It's commonly used in fried or battered dishes. Just like all the other fish on this list, wild Alaskan pollock contains a wide range of nutrients, which makes it an amazing addition to your diet.

Since fish is one of the main sources of protein on the Pesco-Mediterranean diet, you should learn how to cook it in different ways. Fortunately, there are many options to do this like steaming, poaching, broiling, grilling, and even air frying. As you follow this healthy diet, you will learn how to appreciate different types of fish along with all of the health benefits they have to offer.

## The Most Nutrient-Dense Seafood

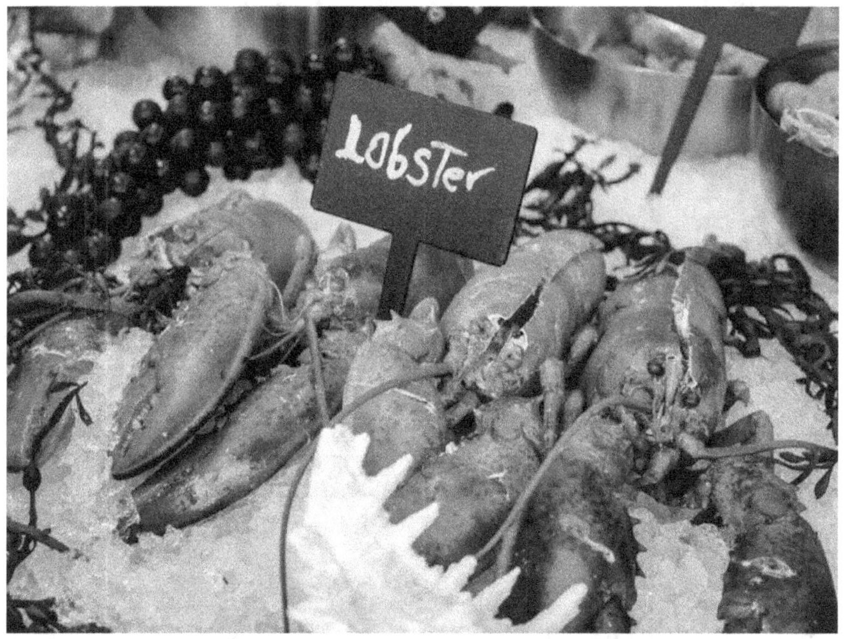


Apart from fish, your main source of protein would be different types of seafood. The Pesco-Mediterranean diet is all about lean and healthy protein sources. Since there are many varieties of fish and seafood to choose from, this makes the diet highly sustainable and enjoyable. When it comes to seafood, here are some of the healthiest options you can eat:

- **Abalone**

This shellfish offers a number of beneficial nutrients like protein and omega-3 fatty acids while being low-fat. Abalone is also an excellent iodine source. It has a chewy, soft texture with a taste that's savory and creamy.

- **Clams**

This is another type of shellfish that offers incredible nutritional value. They are exceptionally rich in vitamin B12. As part of the mollusk family, clams are soft and chewy with a salty taste. You can eat clams on their own after seasoning them lightly or you can add them to soups, stews, and other dishes.

- **Crab**

Surprisingly, crab is low-calorie seafood that has high nutritional value. It contains several vitamins, minerals, protein, and omega-3 fatty acids. The texture of crab meat is similar to white fish and it has a subtle, sweet flavor. Although many people are allergic to crab (you may want to observe yourself first), this is amazing food to add to your diet.

- **Eel**

This seafood might look like a snake but it's actually a type of fish. Eel is more popular in Asian countries, which is too bad because it has an incredible nutritional profile. Apart from omega-3s, eels contain other healthy nutrients like zinc, iron, magnesium, calcium, and more.

- **Lobster**

Although expensive, you should try to add more lobster to your diet as this shellfish is extremely nutritious. Lobster is high in protein and other essential nutrients despite being low in calories. However, like crab, this seafood commonly causes allergic reactions in a lot of people.

- **Mussels**

This shellfish belongs to a mollusk family and it offers a number of health benefits. Mussels are rich in manganese and B-vitamins. They also contain a good amount of omega-3, which is why mussels are considered healthy. These mollusks have a chewy, soft texture and a mildly salty taste. You can season mussels and eat them on their own or add them to various dishes for a nutritional boost.

- **Octopus**

This seafood isn't very common in Western cuisine but it is becoming more popular. In Asian and Mediterranean countries, octopus is an important part of their diets. It's quite tricky to cook octopus but once you get the hang of it, you can enjoy its high omega-3 and other heart-healthy benefits.

- **Oysters**

These shellfish may have a slimy appearance and texture, but they are one of the healthiest types of seafood you can eat. In fact, oysters are almost as nutrient-dense as liver, gizzard, and other organ meats. You can eat oysters raw or you can cook them too. They contain B-vitamins, copper, zinc, and vitamin D, which is quite rare.

- **Scallops**

A lot of people feel intimidated when cooking scallops, especially because they are very easy to overcook. But just like octopus, if you get the hang of cooking scallops perfectly, you can enjoy their taste along with the many brain and health-boosting nutrients they contain.

- **Seaweed**

Sea veggies like seaweed are another remarkable group of seafood you should include in your Pesco-Mediterranean diet. Apart from containing a wide range of nutrients, seaweed also contains a number of unique compounds that are beneficial to your health. Seaweed is rich in iron and there are many varieties to choose from including wakame, nori, kelp, and kombu.

- **Shrimp**

This crustacean is an excellent source of protein, healthy fats, choline, selenium, and other micronutrients. It's very quick and easy to cook shrimp and it's extremely versatile too. You can even use shrimp in kid-friendly dishes because of its appealing taste and texture. This crustacean is also rich in iron and zinc while being low in calories.

- **Squid**

Also called calamari, this is one of the most popular types of seafood in the world. You can prepare squid in different ways and some people even eat it raw. Squid is another excellent option as it contains a number of essential minerals and vitamins to help improve your health.

With all of these seafood options and more, your Pesco-Mediterranean diet just keeps becoming more and more varied. But there is more to look forward to as this diet allows you to eat the healthiest foods on the planet without having to resort to eating the same things over and over again.

# Chapter 7:

# Nuts, Seeds, and Healthy Oils

Nuts belong to the Pesco-Mediterranean diet because they contain a wide range of nutrients. Most nuts contain healthy oils too. They are also very versatile as you can eat them raw, cook them, or use them in different kinds of dishes. Studies have shown that adding nuts to your diet can help protect you against diabetes, heart disease, and other chronic conditions. Seeds are also a must-have on this diet. Aside from consuming seeds whole, you can consume seed oils, which contain all the nutrients of whole seeds too.

You can include different types of nuts and seeds in your diet to make you healthy and strong. Each seed and nut has its own nutrient content so consuming different varieties will definitely make your meals more nutritious. For instance, instead of snacking on a sweet pastry, you can take a handful of nuts or seeds to make you feel full and satisfied. Just try to avoid salted or sweetened nuts as these will add unnecessary sugar and salt to your diet. Even though the Pesco-Mediterranean diet isn't exclusively plant-based, nuts and seeds are an excellent addition to it.

Speaking of a valuable addition to your diet, fats belong to this category too. Fats are an essential part of your diet and you shouldn't be scared of them. One of the most common beliefs is that consuming fats leads to weight gain, but this isn't always true. Your body needs fat to function well. If you want to benefit from fat instead of compromising your health because of it, focus on healthy fats. When choosing fats and oils, think about the dishes you are planning to make. Some oils may offer a lot of nutrients, but they aren't ideal for cooking. In the same way, some oils are great for cooking, but they don't contain the nutrients you need to stay healthy. To help you decide, here is a quick guide:

- For baking, choose a neutral oil like coconut oil that won't interfere with the flavors of your dish.
- For dressings, choose a flavorful oil like flaxseed or olive oil.
- For frying, choose a neutral oil with a high smoking point like grapeseed oil so you don't end up burning your food.
- For searing or sautéing, choose a flavorful oil with a low smoking point like sesame oil.

You should also remember that different oils offer different benefits. Later, we will discuss this further. But for now, let's take a look at all the good things nuts, seeds, and healthy fats have to offer, which is why they belong to the Pesco-Mediterranean diet.

## How Do Nuts, Seeds, and Healthy Oils Benefit Your Health?

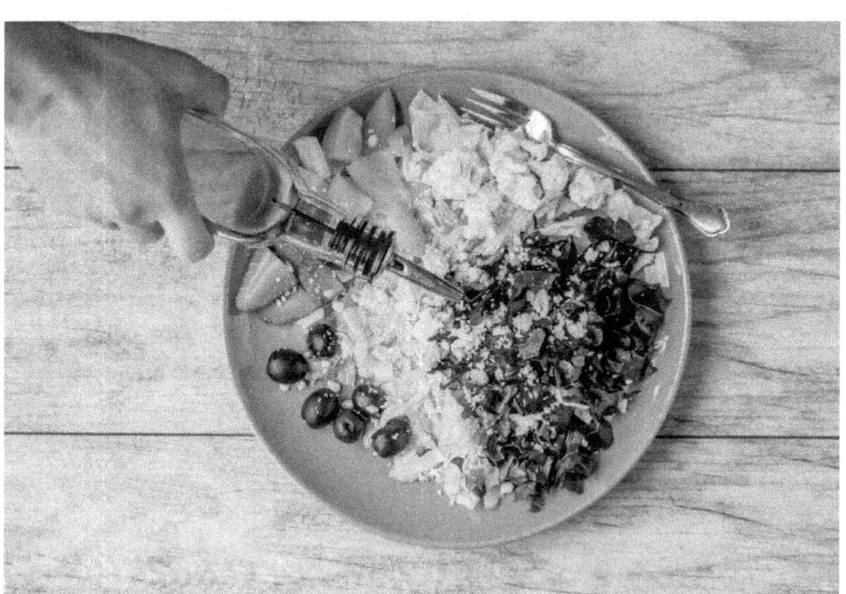

Adding nuts, seeds, and healthy fats to your meals will truly make you a follower of the Pesco-Mediterranean diet. If you do research, you will discover that a lot of Mediterranean dishes contain these ingredients. Of course, the flavor isn't the only thing that nuts, seeds, and healthy fats contribute to your meals. To give you a better idea of why these foods are essential to your diet, let's go through their benefits:

## *Nuts and Seeds*

Nuts and seeds are very hugely beneficial to your diet because they contain a lot of nutrients. If you aren't a big fan of nuts or seeds, here are the advantages of these foods you can enjoy:

- **Rich in essential nutrients**

   Most nuts are excellent sources of vitamin B2, vitamin E, protein, fiber, folate, phosphorus, copper, selenium, potassium, copper, magnesium, and other essential nutrients. They also have a superb omega-3 fatty acid profile. Nuts are rich in linolenic and linoleic acids, two types of essential fatty acids. Although nuts are high in fat too, these are typically unsaturated fats, which offer a number of health benefits. Apart from having beneficial nutrients, nuts are also low on the glycemic index. This means that they are ideal for people who suffer from type 2 diabetes and other issues with insulin resistance.

- **Promotes the health of your heart**

   Regular consumption of nuts can promote the health of your heart. This is mainly because of the protein, unsaturated fats, phytochemicals, and fiber content of different nuts. Nuts are excellent sources of polyunsaturated and monounsaturated fats, which help lower your LDL cholesterol levels. This is a huge advantage since LDL cholesterol contributes to the accumulation of plaque within your arteries. When this happens, the passageways of your arteries become narrow and this may result in coronary heart disease. Aside from this benefit, nuts also help maintain the health of your blood vessels while regulating your blood pressure levels. This is thanks to the arginine content of nuts. Since nuts are also high in antioxidants, they also offer anti-inflammatory benefits.

- **Helps you maintain a healthy weight**

Even though nuts are high in healthy fats, this doesn't mean that eating them will cause you to gain weight—unless you frequently overindulge in them. But if you eat the right types of nuts and in the right quantities, this can even help you shed those stubborn excess pounds. Nuts are a common ingredient in diets that promote weight loss. They are especially effective in promoting fat loss in the lower abdominal region. This helps prevent the development of chronic diseases like diabetes and heart disease. Nuts also help with your body's regulatory processes in the following ways:

  - Eating nuts promotes fullness, which means that you will reduce your food intake without even trying. This benefit comes from the high fiber and protein contents of nuts.
  - Since the fat content of nuts isn't fully digested by your body, this means that your body won't absorb a lot of fat.
  - Consuming nuts may also help your body burn more energy. This means that your body won't store any excess fat so you won't gain weight.

Collectively, all of these benefits will help you lose weight and maintain a healthy weight once you reach it. And when you combine these nuts with all the other healthy foods on the

Pesco-Mediterranean diet, you will surely achieve your target weight along with all your other health goals.

## *Healthy Fats*

As you now know, fats are an essential part of a healthy diet. In particular, healthy fats are the ones you should be adding to your diet. Here are some of the benefits of healthy fats:

- **Provides anti-inflammatory properties**

  You can enjoy this particular benefit from natural oils like avocado, olive, walnut, and flaxseed. Natural oils have intrinsic anti-inflammatory benefits that come from specific compounds they contain. For instance, olive oil and extra-virgin olive oil contain a compound called oleocanthal, which has anti-inflammatory effects. Also, the monounsaturated fatty acid content of olive oil can be used by the body to ease inflammation and reduce the adverse effects of inflammatory conditions like arthritis and asthma.

- **Promotes cardiovascular health**

  This is one benefit that healthy fats shares with nuts and seeds. Certain oils contain monounsaturated, polyunsaturated, and unsaturated fats, which can help reduce your risk of heart disease and all of its associated factors. Healthy fats boost your HDL cholesterol levels while lowering your LDL cholesterol levels. When these happen, they will give your heart health a boost.

- **Highly versatile**

Finally, healthy fats and oils are amazingly versatile, which means that you can use them in different dishes on the Pesco-Mediterranean diet. You can use these oils for cooking, drizzling, dipping, and more. As mentioned, the oil you choose will depend on how you plan to use it. One thing's for sure, no matter how you plan to use oil in your meals, you will always have a couple of options to choose from.

Knowing all of these benefits will surely make you feel more excited to add nuts, seeds, and healthy fats to your diet. Now, it's time for you to learn which are the best options to incorporate into your new eating pattern.

## The Most Beneficial Nuts and Seeds

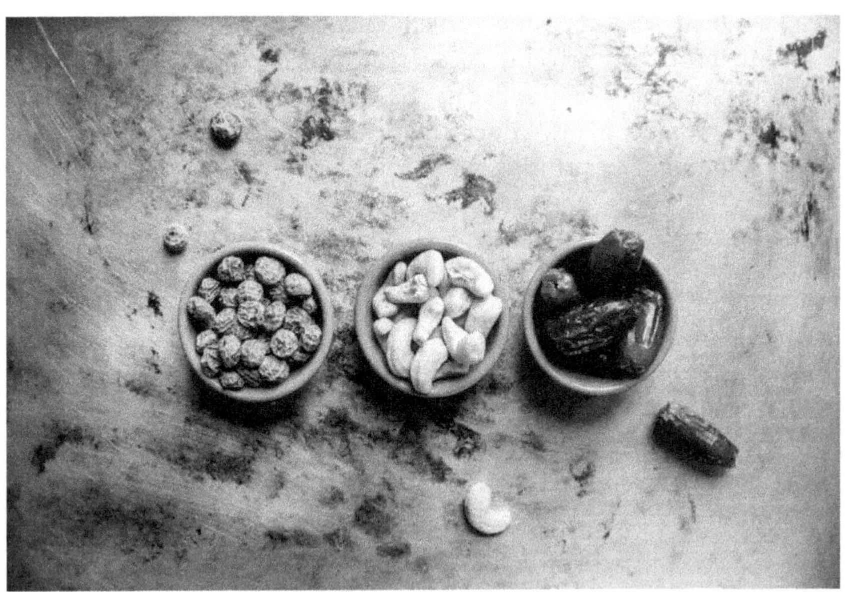

By following the Pesco-Mediterranean diet, you will be increasing your consumption of plant-based foods. Fortunately, there are so many different types of plant-based foods to choose from, all of which add more nutrients and flavors to your meals. Now that you know all of the benefits of nuts and seeds, it's time to discuss the healthiest options to add to your diet. These include:

- **Almonds**

    These nuts are very popular as they are used in a wide range of dishes and desserts. As a follower of the Pesco-Mediterranean diet, you should incorporate almonds into your diet as they are chock-full of fiber, protein, manganese, magnesium, phosphorus, riboflavin, copper, and vitamin E.

    Apart from adding almonds to recipes, you can also eat a handful of these flavorful nuts as a snack. Eat them on their own or pair them with a piece of fruit for a healthy and satisfying snack. These nuts also contain the most calcium among all nuts. By adding almonds to your diet, you can combat inflammation, improve your heart health, and even lose weight.

- **Brazil nuts**

    These nuts contain the essential mineral selenium, which is beneficial to your immune system, reproductive health, and thyroid function. Eat one or two Brazil nuts each day to increase your selenium levels. Just don't eat more than that as too much selenium can cause adverse effects like hair loss, diarrhea, or brittle nails.

- **Cashews**

    These nuts are an excellent source of iron, magnesium, copper, and other healthy nutrients. By adding these nuts to your diet, you can increase your antioxidant intake, which improves your immunity.

- **Chia seeds**

We have already discussed the importance of chia seeds in Chapter 4, which focused on fiber. Apart from being high in fiber, this superfood also contains high levels of antioxidants and omega-3 fatty acids, both of which are very beneficial. Chia seeds are also high in magnesium, folate, calcium, and iron. These seeds improve the health of your bones, promote heart health, and reduce your triglyceride levels.

- **Cucumber seeds**

Although you might not think of eating the seeds of cucumbers, you should start doing so. These tiny seeds offer several health benefits as they contain various nutrients that support your health such as flavonoids and carotenoids. The best thing about cucumber seeds is that you can get them from cucumbers, a veggie that is readily available everywhere. When using cucumbers in salads or other dishes, don't remove the seeds. In fact, you should scoop up any seeds that fall on your plate whenever you eat cucumbers!

- **Flaxseeds**

When ground, these seeds can be used as a substitute for eggs when baking. But you can also sprinkle ground flaxseeds over oatmeal, soup, and other dishes to give your meals a boost of omega-3s and fiber. It's more beneficial to consume ground or milled flax seeds because the whole seeds tend to pass through the body without being digested. This means that you won't get the nutritional benefits they offer because your body cannot break them down.

Flaxseeds have a nutty flavor, which is why they're more commonly added in sweet recipes. These super seeds help lower your LDL cholesterol level, reduce your risk of heart disease, stabilize your blood sugar levels, and even promote the health of your eyes and brain. Flaxseeds also contain a type of estrogen known as lignans that help in the prevention of cancer.

- **Pistachios**

These savory nuts are high in an amino acid known as arginine, which helps improve the flow of blood in your body. This promotes the health of your heart and it also helps with leg cramps, hypertension, and similar conditions. Among all nuts, pistachios have the lowest amount of fat and calories. They are also high in manganese, vitamin B6, and copper, all of which are heart-healthy. When choosing pistachios, opt for those with natural-colored shells or those which have already been shelled. Use pistachios as a crust for baked fish, as a topping for salads, or as a nutritious snack.

- **Pumpkin seeds**

These seeds are extremely healthy as they are high in protein, iron, zinc, magnesium, and vitamin B. Pumpkin seeds also contain tryptophan, a type of amino acid that can help reduce feelings of anxiety.

- **Quinoa**

This is another healthy option that we have already discussed, this time in Chapter 5, which focused on legumes and whole grains. Technically, quinoa is a type of seed even though it is typically treated as a whole grain in various recipes. Quinoa is considered a complete protein as it contains all of the essential amino acids. It also has a low glycemic index, which means eating meals that contain quinoa won't cause extreme spikes in your levels of blood glucose. This versatile seed is easy to prepare and you can use it in both sweet and savory dishes. You can also have it as a side dish along with a healthy protein like salmon or lobster.

- **Sesame seeds**

These seeds are chock-full of magnesium and protein. Sesame seeds also contain good amounts of omega-6 fatty acids, zinc, and iron. Sprinkle sesame seeds on salads, veggie dishes, or baked goods. You can also use sesame seeds to make a seed butter known as tahini. Then you can use this in various dips, dressings, and dishes.

- **Walnuts**

Although some people don't consider walnuts as the tastiest nuts, they are incredibly nutritious. Walnuts contain high amounts of antioxidants, which help combat damage caused by free radicals. Compared to other nuts, walnuts also contain higher amounts of omega-3s, the healthy and beneficial fat. In particular, walnuts are rich in plant-based omega-3 fatty acid known as alpha-linolenic acid or ALA. Walnuts also contain phosphorus, fiber, proteins, and magnesium. These healthy nuts are considered a superfood as they help in weight management, they promote heart health, and they offer anti-inflammatory benefits too.

These are just some examples of the healthiest nuts and seeds to add to your Pesco-Mediterranean diet—there are many more. Add more nuts and seeds to your dishes to boost your nutrition and enjoy their numerous health benefits.

# The Most Beneficial Healthy Oils

To increase your chances of success on the Pesco-Mediterranean diet, you should learn how to prepare and cook your own meals. While whipping up different types of dishes, you will need various oils for cooking and making everything more flavorful. Oils are an excellent way to add healthy fats to your diet. When choosing oils, opt for the healthiest ones including:

- **Avocado oil**

  This oil is low in saturated fats and high in monounsaturated fats, which are good for the heart. Now that more people are becoming interested in healthy foods, avocado oil has become wildly popular. This oil has neutral and delicate flavors and a high smoke point. Although avocado oil is one of the more expensive oils, it is an amazingly healthy option for you. Just make sure to keep your avocado oil in a dark, hidden place as it tends to oxidize easily in bright light. One great thing about avocado oil is that you can also use it on your skin. Since this oil is rich in vitamin E, it helps reduce the common signs of aging while making your skin softer too.

- **Coconut oil**

  The great thing about this oil is that it naturally contains saturated fats that elevate your levels of HDL cholesterol while transforming your LDL cholesterol to make it less harmful. The main health benefit of coconut oil is that it promotes heart health. However, when it comes to coconut oil, there are conflicting opinions. Although this is a plant-based oil, some people are concerned with its high saturated fat content. Probably the best way to get the most out of this oil is by using it occasionally so you don't go overboard.

- **Flaxseed oil**

Also known as linseed oil, this is rich in ALA, which helps in the prevention of strokes and heart attacks. Flaxseed oil also contains omega-6s that promote the health of your skin. Just like avocado oil, this oil tends to get compromised, but this time, when it's exposed to heat. Therefore, it's best to store your flaxseed oil in the refrigerator. Purchase this oil from health food stores to make sure that you're getting high-quality food-grade oil without any added chemicals. It's also important to note that this oil cannot be used for cooking. Instead, you can drizzle it over dips and dressings to add more nutrition and an interesting flavor to your dishes.

- **Grapeseed oil**

This oil is the perfect option for low-fat diets since it spreads easily, which means that you won't have to use a lot, especially when adding it to salads. Grapeseed oil is suitable for cooking (even frying) because it isn't as volatile as other vegetable oils. However, this oil won't add much flavor to your dishes so you may have to use herbs, spices, and other healthy seasonings to make your meals more flavorful.

- **Olive oil**

Among all oils, this is one of the healthiest and most popular. Olive oil lowers your LDL cholesterol levels while raising your HDL cholesterol levels, which means that it offers heart-health benefits. Compared to other types of natural oils, olive oil contains higher amounts of monounsaturated fats. It even helps calm stomach ulcers. You can use olive oil in different types of dishes and you can also use it for cooking. Just be careful when cooking with this oil as its taste and nutritional profile can change when you exceed its smoking point.

One variation of olive oil is extra-virgin olive oil, which is more flavorful and contains more monounsaturated fats than pure olive oil. Other than that, it shares the same benefits as olive oil. However, you cannot use this type for roasting and frying because of its lower smoking point. Still, either of these options would be an amazing addition to your Pesco-Mediterranean diet.

- **Peanut oil**

When it comes to flavorful oils, this is a great choice. However, this can also be its weakness as you should only use peanut oil for cooking if you want to add a peanut flavor to your dishes. This makes it a healthy oil for sautéing, stir-frying, and making dishes with a nutty flavor. Peanut oil is low in saturated fats and it's a good source of vitamin E. Since it also has a high smoking point, you can use it for frying too.

- **Pumpkin seed oil**

This oil is chock-full of omega-3, omega-6, and zinc making it beneficial for your reproductive and immune systems. Pumpkin seed oil can even help ease inflammation in those who suffer from arthritis. Healthy and flavorful as this oil is, it's not a great choice for cooking. The reason for this is that heating pumpkin seed oil tends to reduce its nutritional value. Instead, drizzle it over dishes like mashed potato, salads, or risotto to make your dishes look and taste better.

- **Safflower oil**

This is a flavorless oil that is rich in linoleic acid, which helps combat heart disease. Even though many types of vegetable oils are considered unhealthy, this is one of the few exceptions. It's low in saturated fats, it has a high smoking point, and it is also rich in omega-9 fatty acids. You can either get monounsaturated safflower oil for cooking or polyunsaturated safflower oil for drizzling or topping over sauces, salads, and other dishes.

- **Sesame oil**

This oil is incredibly flavorful and it's another healthy option on the Pesco-Mediterranean diet. Because of its strong flavor, a little bit goes a long way. If you're allergic to peanuts, you can use sesame oil as an alternative to your dishes. This is a cold-pressed oil that also happens to be unrefined.

- **Walnut oil**

With its low smoking point, this oil isn't ideal for cooking. But the good news is, walnut oil isn't just healthy and flavorful. You can also use it in different ways. For instance, you can drizzle walnut oil over desserts, pancakes, and even fresh fruits to add more health and flavor. Walnut oil contains a good amount of omega-3 and omega-6 fatty acids, which have anti-inflammatory benefits.

Since healthy oils and fats are essential in flavoring your dishes on the Pesco-Mediterranean diet, you can use these options while cooking or preparing your meals. You can also learn more about and experiment with other healthy oils to add to your diet.

Chapter 8:

# The Good and Bad Sides of the Pesco-Mediterranean Diet

Although the Pesco-Mediterranean diet is the ideal diet for overall health, it's not considered a 'perfect' diet. It offers a number of incredible benefits, but it also comes with its own set of precautions. For you to really understand this diet, it's important for you to know both sides. Only knowing the good things about a diet can lead to disastrous results. For instance, if you choose to follow a diet that is purely plant-based because you read several resources that raved about it, you won't know the possible risks like not getting enough of certain nutrients. This can be very dangerous to your health, especially if the nutrient deficiency you develop will start taking a toll on your body. Therefore, in this chapter, we will focus on the good and (the potential) bad sides of the Pesco-Mediterranean diet. This will give you a complete picture of what this diet is all about before we move on to the final part of this book—combining it with intermittent fasting.

# Maintaining a Healthy Weight for the Long-Run

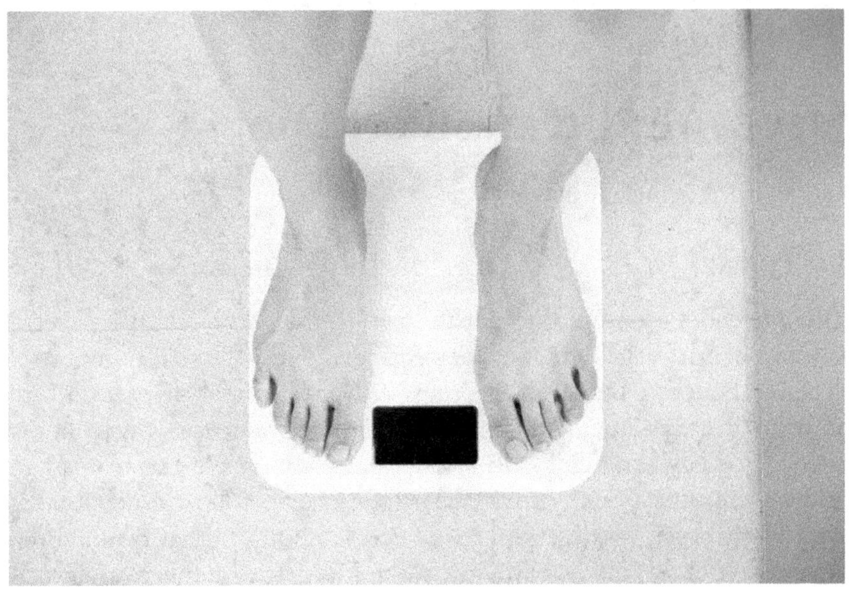

One of the most important benefits of the Pesco-Mediterranean diet is that it can help you lose weight. By nature, this diet encourages you to eat healthier. By avoiding red meat and processed food from your diet, you will be taking away the main food sources that tend to cause unhealthy weight gain. Several studies have shown that overweight and obese people who follow the Mediterranean diet lose more weight compared to those who follow low-carb or low-fat diets. This effect can also be observed in people who follow the Pescatarian diet.

Probably the main reason for this is the types of food eaten on both diets. As you know, the focus of these diets is on fruits, vegetables, whole grains, fish, seafood, and healthy fats. These foods are not only healthy, but they are all naturally filling. This means that you will always feel full, satiated, and happy after every meal. Another reason why these diets (and the Pesco-Mediterranean diet combination) are so effective is that you won't focus on caloric restriction. For a lot of people, especially those who are struggling with their weight, following a restrictive diet tends to make them feel worse about themselves. Then they end up focusing on food too much, which often results in deciding to give up. When they go back to their old eating habits, they tend to regain all the weight they have lost—and then some.

But the Pesco-Mediterranean diet offers a different solution. It will help you lose those stubborn excess pounds while still being able to enjoy flavorful, satisfying, and nutrient-rich meals and snacks. This makes it more sustainable in the long-term. And once you have achieved your target weight, you can maintain that weight by continuing with the Pesco-Mediterranean diet.

Even if you are on the other end of the spectrum—if you are trying to gain weight—this diet can help you out too. As you plan your dishes, all you have to do is either increase your portions or add more ingredients to your meals. For instance, if you have planned to enjoy whole-grain toast with sardines and tomatoes for breakfast, you can add more calories to this dish by adding a few avocado slices. The avocado slices will make the dish healthier, more satisfying, and higher in calories. Continue doing this until you reach a healthy weight then you can gradually go back to the 'normal' portions.

For this benefit, the bottom line is this. The Pesco-Mediterranean diet is the ideal way of eating to help you achieve a healthy weight for life in a natural way. As long as you plan your meals well and learn how to listen to your body, this amazing diet can help you manage your weight. This is one of the greatest benefits of the Pesco-Mediterranean diet, but it's not the only one. Because of the nature of this extraordinary diet combination, there are many other advantages you can look forward to. Let's discuss these next...

## Other Benefits of the Pesco-Mediterranean Diet

For a lot of people, choosing the right diet is a huge challenge. Ultimately, the diet you choose would depend on your health goals. The great thing about the Pesco-Mediterranean diet is that you can follow it no matter what your health goals are. This is because it is not just a diet that will make your heart healthier. It offers so much more. Since this diet is composed of the pescatarian diet and the Mediterranean diet combined, this means that you will get the combined benefits of both diets too. Here are the benefits you can look forward to when you start following the Pesco-Mediterranean diet:

- **Increases your consumption of essential nutrients**

Now that you know how simple the Pesco-Mediterranean diet is, you might still be feeling surprised at how healthy it is. Since this diet encourages you to focus on whole, healthy foods, you will be increasing your consumption of essential nutrients. To do this, you won't have to come up with a strict or extreme plan for your meals. Instead, you will simply teach yourself to make healthier food choices by refocusing your energy on plant-rich foods and fish and seafood for your animal-based proteins. The most important and beneficial nutrients you will get more of on this diet include:

- By focusing on fish and seafood as your main protein source, you get nutrients like zinc, calcium, vitamin B12, and high-quality protein. These are some nutrients you might not get enough of on a purely plant-based diet.
- Apart from fish and seafood, many of the plant-based foods on this diet contain high-quality plant proteins, which are essential to your health too.
- Most of the food options on the Pesco-Mediterranean diet are rich in omega-3 fatty acids. This is a type of healthy fat that helps improve the different aspects of your health.
- By eating both animal and plant-based sources, you are giving yourself the choice of consuming a wide

range of vitamins, minerals, and essential nutrients. And if you add a lot of variety to your diet, this means that you will be nourishing your body with various nutrients too. This, in turn, provides the next few benefits this diet has to offer.

- ### Promotes brain health

There is evidence that shows that the Mediterranean diet, which is half of the Pesco-Mediterranean diet can help improve your memory and overall brain functions. This is mainly thanks to the foods that contain omega-3 fatty acids along with all the other nutrients that can be found in whole foods.

- ### The ideal diet for your heart

In Chapter 2, we discussed the most significant study conducted about the Pesco-Mediterranean diet, which showed that heart health is one of the most important benefits of this diet. Several studies have been done about the pescatarian diet and the Mediterranean diet separately and they have also identified heart health as one of the benefits. This consistency solidifies the claim that the Pesco-Mediterranean diet is ideal for heart health.

This benefit mainly comes from the fact that you will be minimizing or avoiding the consumption of red meat and processed foods. Instead, you will focus on heart-healthy foods like fish, fruits, vegetables, and healthy fats. Also, the weight loss and the protective benefits of this diet will contribute to the improvement of your heart. And if you can pair this with other healthy lifestyle habits like regular exercise and getting enough sleep, you will definitely enjoy this benefit!

- **Strengthens your bones**

Another nutrient you will get a lot of in this diet is calcium. Consuming high amounts of calcium will help make your bones stronger, which reduces your risk of getting fractures even if you fall down.

- **Helps you sleep better**

As your body becomes healthier on the inside, you will also notice yourself being able to sleep better each night. This is an excellent benefit since sleep allows your body to rest, recuperate, and repair itself. When this happens, you become even healthier.

- **Prevents the development of chronic diseases**

With all of the previous benefits mentioned, this good effect is only natural. As your body becomes healthier and stronger, this reduces your risk of developing a number of chronic diseases. One important reason for this is that you won't be eating processed foods as often as before. These foods contain free radicals and other chemicals that can have negative effects on your body. By gradually eliminating processed foods from your diet and replacing these with whole foods, you can potentially avoid the following:

  - By losing weight and maintaining a healthy weight, you reduce your risk of obesity.
  - By consuming foods that have a low glycemic index, you avoid spikes in your blood sugar levels. This is one factor that helps reduce your risk of diabetes.

- ○　　　Plant-based foods, fatty fish, and healthy oils help reduce inflammation in your body, which can also prevent high blood pressure, insulin resistance, and conditions like metabolic syndrome.
- ○　　　This nutrient-rich diet can even help you avoid some types of cancer.

- **When combined with intermittent fasting...**

In itself, the Pesco-Mediterranean diet is extremely beneficial. When you combine it with intermittent fasting, you will also give yourself the chance to enjoy the benefits of this trendy eating pattern. Since intermittent fasting involves periods of fasting and periods of eating, you will improve your health even more. This is because, during the times when you will eat, you will be providing your body with the healthiest types of foods that are part of the Pesco-Mediterranean diet.

As you can see, this diet will surely improve your overall health and well-being in different ways. This is why this diet is quickly rising as a star in the health and fitness world as more and more people are discovering how amazing it is.

# Are There Any Potential Risks?

Since the beginning of this book, we have been talking about all the wonderful things this diet has to offer. Now, you might be wondering if the Pesco-Mediterranean diet is too good to be true or if it has some mind-blowing risks you should be aware of. Here's more good news for you—this diet doesn't have a lot of downsides. It simply has a number of potential drawbacks, which you can easily overcome as long as you are aware of them. These potential downsides include the following:

- Some types of fish, especially the bigger ones like king mackerel, tilefish, or shark may contain high levels of mercury and other toxins. Because of this, you may want to minimize your consumption of these fish. If you are either pregnant or breastfeeding, you may want to avoid these fish for the time being.

- In some cases, people don't realize that they are consuming excess carbs because they focus on starchy veggies, fruits, and even grains. To avoid this, try to balance the dishes you eat through meal planning.

- In the same way, eating excessively high quantities of nuts, olive oils, and other fats might cause you to gain weight. If one of your main goals is to lose weight, this will make you frustrated. Again, meal planning will be a big help as you will learn how to find the right balance at every meal.

Finally, you may struggle if this diet is very different from your current diet, especially at the beginning. The best way to overcome this is by taking things slow and making changes at your own pace. Remember, it's better to make small but consistent changes in your diet rather than doing too much, too fast, which might make you give up after only a few weeks. By keeping all of these in mind, you can start planning your diet transition and focusing on the positive sides of the Pesco-Mediterranean diet.

**Chapter 9:**

# All About Intermittent Fasting

Whether you're into health trends and diets or not, you have probably heard the term, 'fasting' before—and you probably know what it means already. Fasting simply means going for a certain period of time without eating anything. For stricter fasts, you won't even drink anything, not even water! In medical terms and for medical purposes, fasting usually lasts between 8 to 12 hours. But for intermittent fasting, your fasting window can either be shorter or longer.

Fasting is an eating pattern wherein you cycle between periods of fasting and periods of eating. There are different ways to fast intermittently. The main difference between these fasting periods is the duration of their fasting periods. Weight loss is one of the main benefits of fasting. In fact, this is a natural effect because you tend to eat less food when you fast, especially if you have long fasting windows. However, unlike restrictive diets, fasting doesn't focus on caloric restriction. It also doesn't focus on what you should be eating. Instead, intermittent fasting—or IF for short—focuses on when you eat. This is why IF is considered an eating pattern instead of a diet.

Although there are no restrictions on the type or amount of food you can consume during your feasting window (the time when you are allowed to eat), you should still focus on eating healthy foods. This is especially true if you want to get all of the benefits of this healthy eating pattern. Also, since you will be restricting your calories without even trying, it's best to focus on whole, nutrient-dense foods to avoid developing any kind of nutrient deficiencies.

Another amazing benefit of IF is that it gives your digestive system time to rest and repair itself. Digestion involves a lot of work and if you continue eating throughout the day, most of the energy you get goes into this process. But if you regularly provide your digestive system with time to rest through intermittent fasting, this helps improve its health. In line with this, IF also forces your body into a metabolic state known as ketosis. This happens when your digestive system has already broken down all of the food you have eaten. Since you are fasting, you won't be eating anything else. When your body doesn't have any more food to break down, it starts burning your fat stores. This is one reason why weight loss happens when you fast intermittently. Other general benefits of IF include:

- Hormonal regulation.
- Improved insulin sensitivity.
- Protection against certain conditions like type 2 diabetes, cardiovascular disease, cognitive decline, and even cancer.
- Increases metabolism and energy levels.
- Helps slow down the effects and signs of aging.
- Offers protective effects on your genes.

While it's true that IF is extremely beneficial to your health, you must first decide which fasting method to use before you can start. By choosing the right fasting method to combine with your diet (which, in this case, is the Pesco-Mediterranean diet), you can unlock all of the potential benefits of this amazing eating pattern.

# The Various Intermittent Fasting Methods

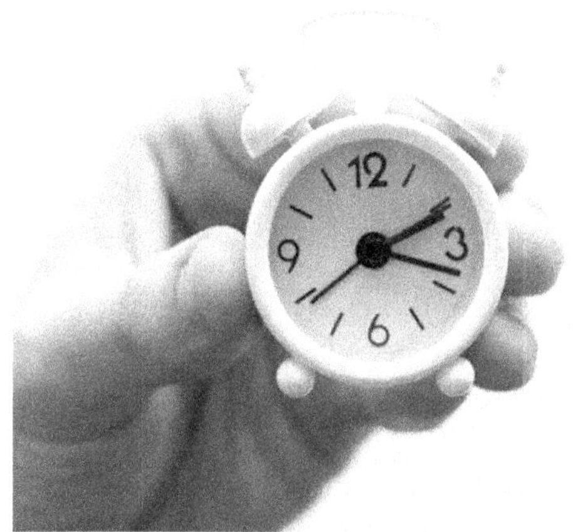

These days, intermittent fasting is a huge trend. People all over the world have started their own IF journey to improve their health, lose weight, or reach their own personal health goals. Since IF works with different types of diets, even the Pesco-Mediterranean diet, you should learn the different fasting methods. That way, you can choose the best method to suit your own needs and lifestyle. The most common IF methods include:

## *5:2 Method*

This is one of the simplest IF methods and it's quite popular too. For the 5:2 method, you would eat normally for five days each week, which means that you will consume regular Pesco-Mediterranean-friendly meals during these days. On the other two days, you will restrict your caloric intake to only 500 calories for women or 600 calories for men. Michael Mosley, a journalist from Britain popularized this method, which is also known as the "Fast Diet."

Since you will only be eating a few calories for two days, you should plan your meals well. For instance, if you're a man, you can consume three 200-calorie meals or two 300-calorie meals throughout the day on your fasting days. Or if you're a woman, you can either consume two 250-calorie meals or two 150-calorie meals and one 100-calorie meal throughout the day on your fasting days. While you are adjusting to this IF method, you may have to count your calories. Once you get the hang of the 5:2 method, you can already plan your meals well without having to count calories.

## 16/8 Method

This method is a bit more intense than the 5:2 method because it involves fasting every day, but it's relatively popular too. For the 16/8 method, you will fast each day for 16 hours and eat your meals for the remaining 8 hours. One variation of this method is the 14/10 method wherein you fast for 14 hours and eat for 10 hours each day. Within your daily feasting window, you can consume your regular meals. Martin Berkhan, the fitness expert popularized this method, which is also called the "Leangains Protocol."

Since this method allows you to eat what you want during your feasting window, many people believe that it's easier than the other methods. This is especially true if you plan your fasting and feasting windows carefully. For instance, if your fasting window starts at 7:00 pm, it will end at 11:00 am the next day. This means that you can have your first meal every 11:00 am and continue eating meals and snacks until 7:00 pm. For such a schedule, it includes the time when you sleep. This makes it much easier because you won't feel hungry while you're sleeping! But in cases where you work at night and sleep during the day, you can easily modify your schedule to make this method work for you.

## Eat-Stop-Eat Method

This method is more flexible than the 5:2 method as you can choose to fast either once or twice each week. It is also more intense as you won't be eating anything for a whole day during your fasting windows. Brad Pilon, another fitness expert, popularized this diet and it has gained a good number of followers in recent years. This is one of the simpler methods as you only have to set a day (or two) and start your fasting window.

For instance, if you have your last meal at 8:00 pm on a Monday and your fasting day is on Tuesday, your next meal will be at 8:00 pm on Tuesday to complete a 24-hour fast. This method can help you lose weight quickly, as long as, you don't try to overcompensate by overeating before or after your fasting days. If you think that this method is too difficult for you (like if you're new to fasting), you may want to start with the 5:2 method first so that you get used to eating fewer calories two days each week before you start fasting for the whole day.

## Alternate-Day Fasting Method

This is another simple method wherein you will fast every other day. Completely fasting on alternate days is a huge challenge for a lot of people, even those who have been following IF for some time. The main downside of this method is feeling extremely hungry 3 to 4 times each week. This is definitely not a pleasant experience, which might cause you to quit after just one or two weeks. If you really want to try this method, you can start with an easier variation wherein you will consume up to 500 calories (for women) or 600 calories (for men) during your fasting days. That way, you won't feel like you are restricting yourself completely several times a week.

### *One Meal a Day Method*

This method is the most intense and extreme among all IF methods and generally, it isn't considered sustainable in the long-run. Ori Hofmekler, the fitness expert, popularized this method and it's also known as the "Warrior Diet." As the name implies, it involves eating just one meal each day. Basically, you will be giving yourself a 4-hour feasting window every day then the other 20 hours would be spent fasting.

An easier variation of this method involves consuming small amounts of raw vegetables and fruits throughout the day then eating a huge meal for dinner. This variation makes the OMAD method more sustainable. Just make sure to consume whole, unprocessed foods every day while following this method. Fortunately, the Pesco-Mediterranean diet encourages you to eat such foods, which means that this method will also work when paired with the Pesco-Mediterranean diet.

### *Overnight Fasting Method*

This is the simplest IF method as it only involves fasting for a period of 12 hours each night. Since you will spend most of this time sleeping, you might not even feel that you are fasting intermittently. This makes the Overnight Fasting method ideal for beginners as it will give your body a chance to adjust to fasting without feeling like you are struggling. If one of your health goals is to lose weight, you may want to reduce your portions too, since this method doesn't maximize the benefits of fasting.

### *Spontaneous Meal Skipping*

This method is even easier as you would only fast when you feel like it. If you're thinking about following IF but you're not yet ready, you can prepare yourself by following this method. Whenever mealtime comes along and you don't feel hungry, you can choose to skip that meal spontaneously. Doing this once in a while allows you to enjoy some benefits of fasting without following a more structured schedule. Just like the Overnight Fasting method, this method gives you a chance to know what it feels like to fast for a certain period of time. Whenever it's convenient for you, you're too busy to eat, or you just don't feel like eating, you can skip your meals to give your digestive system a break.

No matter which IF method you choose, you can drink zero-calorie beverages like plain tea or coffee, or water during your fasting windows. These beverages will keep you hydrated while reducing your feelings of hunger. Also, it's best to stick with your Pesco-Mediterranean diet during your feasting windows. Since this diet focuses on healthy, whole foods, you will be able to nourish your body adequately even if you are reducing your caloric intake through fasting.

# Combining the Pesco-Mediterranean Diet with Intermittent Fasting

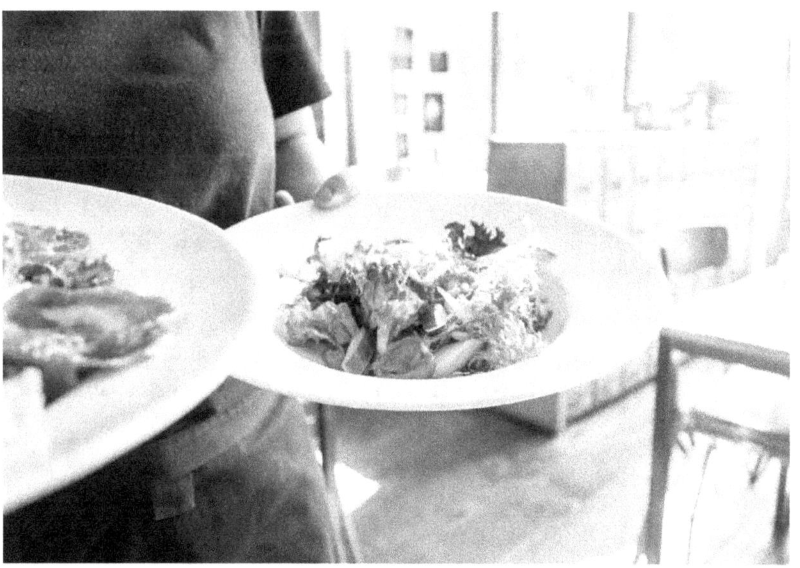

The Pesco-Mediterranean diet is rich in plants, fish, seafood, and healthy fats. In itself, it is already extremely healthy and beneficial. On its own, intermittent fasting also provides a number of health benefits ranging from weight loss to the prevention of chronic diseases. When you combine this eating pattern with the ideal Pesco-Mediterranean diet, you get a winning combination that will improve your health in so many ways.

When paired with IF, the Pesco-Mediterranean diet will provide you with the best results in terms of health improvements, especially your heart health. Among all of the methods mentioned in the last section, the ones that are commonly paired with this diet are the 5:2 and 16/8 method and their variations. For instance, you can choose to eat normally for five days each week then restrict your caloric intake for the other two days, as long as you stick with this diet. Or if you have chosen the 16/8 method, you can set your fasting windows between 8 to 12 hours each day then fast for the remaining hours. Aside from planning the IF method to pair with the Pesco-Mediterranean diet, here are other tips to help you succeed:

- **Focus on whole foods**

Intermittent fasting isn't about the food you eat, but it's more about when you should be eating your meals. But if you want to make the most out of this winning diet-eating pattern combination, you should focus on whole foods all throughout your feasting windows. Of course, this should be a cinch because half of this pairing—the Pesco-Mediterranean diet—is all about whole foods like fruits, vegetables, nuts, seeds, legumes, fish, seafood, olive oil, and so on. By focusing on these foods during your feasting windows, you will provide your body with incredible nourishment while giving your digestive system time to rest during your fasting windows.

- **Remember... water is your friend**

One thing IF and the Pesco-Mediterranean diet have in common is that they both encourage you to drink more water. In fact, for the latter, water is the recommended staple beverage. To make sure you are well-hydrated even during your fasting windows, drink a lot of water. You can flavor your water using fresh fruits and veggies to give your drinks a nutrient boost too. Apart from water, other suitable drinks for this combination are plain coffee or tea. These are healthy options too since they contain antioxidants and other beneficial compounds.

- **Combine the diet and eating plan when you're ready**

The mere thought of starting a new eating pattern and a new diet at the same time may seem overwhelming to you (as it does to a lot of people). The good news is, you don't have to start your Pesco-Mediterranean journey with IF right away. If your current diet is widely different from the Pesco-Mediterranean diet, you can gradually transition into this diet first. Make small changes to your current diet until you get used to the recommended foods and choosing these foods comes more naturally to you.

When you feel like you have already transitioned into the Pesco-Mediterranean diet (even if you are still in the process of transitioning completely) and you feel like you're ready to take things up a notch, you can start incorporating IF into your life. Conversely, you can also start by practicing IF first before shifting to the Pesco-Mediterranean diet. Either way, you will increase your chances of success by going at your own pace. If you feel like you're not yet ready, give yourself more time. This will make it a more positive experience for you.

- **Vary your diet**

The more varied your diet is, the more motivated you will be to stick with it long-term. Think about it: would you want to follow a certain diet if you only allow yourself to eat for four hours each day and you are only allowed to eat the same types of food over and over again? Probably, not.

To make this combination work, variation is key. And here's more good news for you—the Pesco-Mediterranean diet allows you to eat a wide range of whole foods. This means that you can create endless combinations for your meals, snacks, and desserts. Whether you choose to eat out or cook your own meals, you will never run out of options on this diet. This makes it an ideal diet to pair with IF since you will always have interesting choices to eat during your feasting windows.

- **Learn to make friendly and healthy substitutions**

One of the biggest challenges people face when starting a new diet is letting go of their old eating habits. For instance, if you are a huge fan of red meat, giving up beef, pork, lamb, and more can be extremely challenging for you. Instead of being too strict on yourself, learn how to find healthier, Pesco-Mediterranean-friendly substitutions for the food you have to minimize or avoid.

In our example, instead of always eating red meat, why don't you treat yourself to a lobster dinner or a flavorful salmon steak? Training yourself to choose healthier protein sources and eating more plants will take time and effort. But if you can whip up scrumptious dishes for yourself, transitioning into the Pesco-Mediterranean diet will become so much easier and more enjoyable for you. And whenever it's time for you to eat, you will always look forward to your meals. Just remember to...

- **Watch your portions!**

This is very important, especially when you start following IF. During your feasting windows, you should eat as you normally would instead of overeating or overindulging to compensate for the meals you miss during your fasting windows. Remember, one of the main reasons why IF is so effective is that it gives your digestive system a break. But if you consume too much food during your feasting windows, your digestive system will have to work harder to break down everything completely. You don't have to reduce your portions unless you are trying to lose a lot of excess pounds to achieve a healthy weight. Just eat the right portions and you will start experiencing the many benefits this healthy combination has to offer.

- **Take a break whenever you need to**

Finally, if you feel too overwhelmed with combining the Pesco-Mediterranean diet with IF, take a break. This doesn't mean that you should give up on it altogether. Instead, you can allow yourself to indulge in a meal or snack that isn't necessarily Pesco-Mediterranean-friendly once in a while just to satisfy your cravings, especially during your transition phase. In the same way, if you have begun your IF journey and you feel too hungry to do anything else, allow yourself to have a light snack. When you're feeling better, you can go back to your Pesco-Mediterranean diet and the IF method you have chosen.

A huge part of following IF and the Pesco-Mediterranean diet is learning how to listen to your body. If you can learn this, making healthier changes to your diet and lifestyle will seem more effortless to you.

# A 7-Day Sample Meal Plan for Your Pesco-Mediterranean Diet

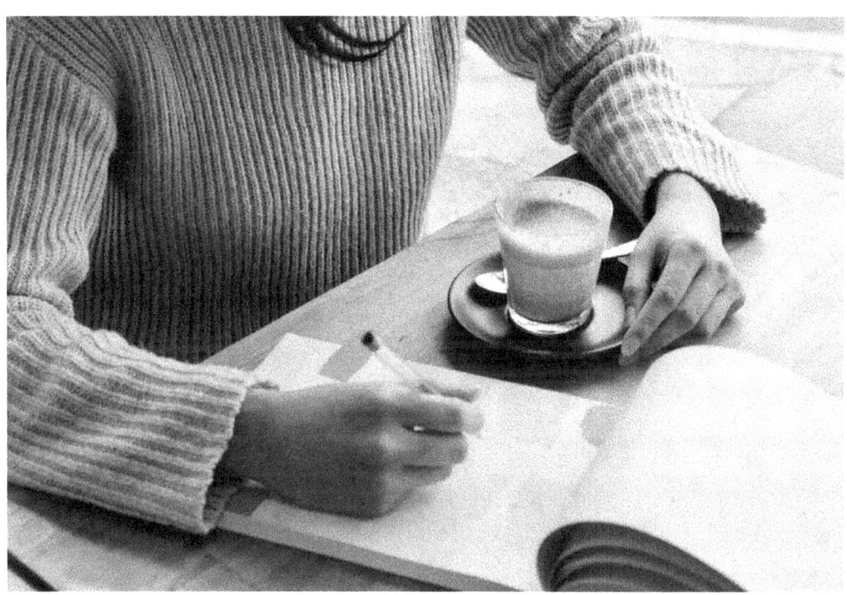

Before we wrap things up, let me share a sample meal plan for you to start with. Meal planning is a smart and convenient way to make your Pesco-Mediterranean diet easier and more fun. By planning your meals beforehand and preparing or cooking everything for the week, you don't have to worry about not having time to create healthy dishes whenever mealtimes come along.

So... what does a typical week on the Pesco-Mediterranean diet look like? Take a look at this meal plan. Since this is just a sample, you can mix and match the meal options according to your own preference.

One word of caution though... you might feel hungry after reading this chapter!

# Day 1

For the first day of your new diet, you can start off with some dishes that are easy and familiar:

- **Breakfast:** Whole-wheat toast with grilled tomatoes and a pan-fried egg. You can also add some avocado slices to make this dish healthier and more filling.
- **Lunch:** A cup of quinoa with sun-dried tomatoes, olives, and bell peppers. You can top this dish with avocado slices or crumbled feta cheese.
- **Dinner:** Half a cup of whole-grain pasta with olive oil, tomato sauce, and grilled veggies. You can top this dish with a tablespoon of Parmesan cheese.
- **Snack (if you get hungry between meals):** Greek yogurt topped with walnuts and blueberries.

# Day 2

For day two, you can start experimenting with more interesting dishes that are suitable for the diet:

- **Breakfast:** A cup of Greek yogurt paired with half a cup of fresh fruits like raspberries, blueberries, or chopped peaches. You can also top this dish with some walnuts or almonds.

- **Lunch:** Two cups of mixed greens with olives and cherry tomatoes drizzled with dressing consisting of vinegar and olive oil. Pair this with whole-grain pita bread and some hummus.

- **Dinner:** A cup of arugula, spinach, or other types of greens with sliced tomatoes and olives. Drizzle with olive oil and toss lightly. Pair this with a small portion of grilled or roasted whitefish.

- **Snack (if you get hungry between meals):** Roasted chickpeas seasoned with thyme and oregano.

# Day 3

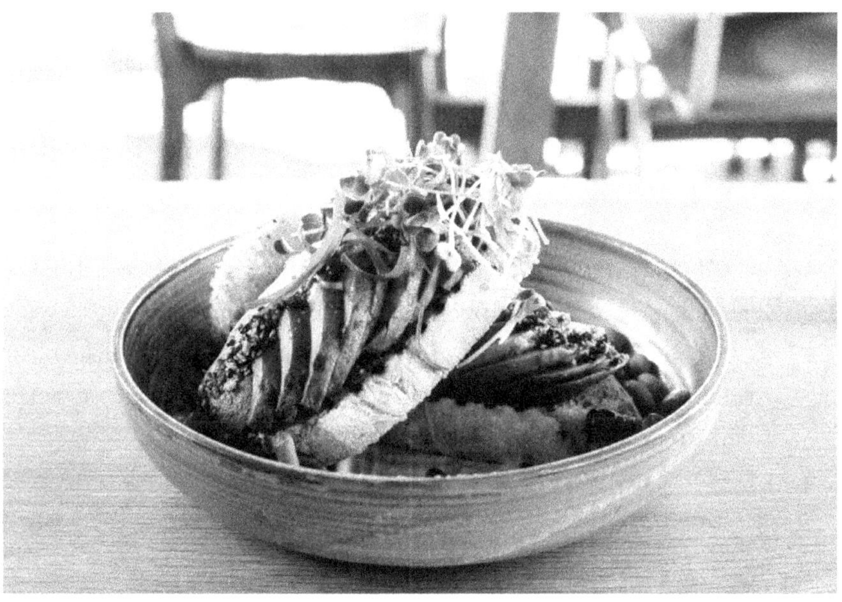

For the third day, continue experimenting with flavorful dishes to help you get used to the rich and healthy style of the Pesco-Mediterranean diet:

- **Breakfast:** Two scrambled eggs with tomatoes, onions, and bell peppers. Top this dish with avocado slices or queso fresco.
- **Lunch:** A whole-grain sandwich with hummus and grilled veggies like onions, bell pepper, zucchini, and eggplant.
- **Dinner:** Oven-roasted veggies like sweet potato, carrots, artichokes, and tomatoes. Season with olive oil and herbs then toss before roasting. Pair this with a cup of whole-grain couscous.
- **Snack (if you get hungry between meals):** Whole fruits like grapes, oranges, or plums.

# Day 4

You're halfway through the week! For the fourth day, you will already have a good idea of what it feels like to follow the Pesco-Mediterranean diet. Just keep going with these dishes:

- **Breakfast:** A cup of Greek yogurt with nuts and berries like almonds, walnuts, blueberries, and raspberries.
- **Lunch:** Whole-grain toast with anchovies roasted in olive oil, and a drizzle of fresh lemon juice. Pair this with a warm salad of steamed tomatoes and kale.
- **Dinner:** A full-sized portion of baked salmon or cod seasoned with black pepper and garlic. Pair this with a small baked potato with chives and olive oil.
- **Snack (if you get hungry between meals):** Fresh veggie sticks with hummus dip.

# Day 5

Now that you're on day five, it's time for some comforting meals to keep you inspired. Give these options a try:

- **Breakfast:** A cup of whole-grain oats sweetened with honey, cinnamon, and dates. You can top this dish with raspberries and shredded almonds or other types of low-sugar fruits.
- **Lunch:** Two cups of mixed greens with tomatoes, cucumber, and olive oil. Pair this with a small portion of roasted shrimp seasoned with salt, pepper, olive oil, and fresh lemon juice.
- **Dinner:** A small whole-grain pizza topped with tomato sauce, grilled veggies, tuna, and low-fat cheese.
- **Snack (if you get hungry between meals):** A handful of dried fruits like figs or apricots.

# Day 6

On the sixth day, you will start feeling more positive about the Pesco-Mediterranean diet because you would have already enjoyed a number of flavorful and healthy recipes for five days. Keep nourishing your body with more dishes like:

- **Breakfast:** Whole-grain toast with goat cheese, queso fresco, ricotta, or some other type of soft cheese. Pair this with chopped figs or blueberries for a touch of sweetness.
- **Lunch:** A cup of white beans boiled with cumin, laurel, and garlic. Pair this with a cup of spinach with cucumber, tomato, crumbled feta cheese, and an olive oil-based dressing.

- **Dinner:** Oven-roasted veggies like zucchini, sweet potato, tomato, carrots, and eggplants. Season with salt, pepper, and olive oil then toss lightly before roasting. Serve with half a cup of quinoa.
- **Snack (if you get hungry between meals):** Baked avocado half with an egg in the middle then seasoned with salt and pepper.

# Day 7

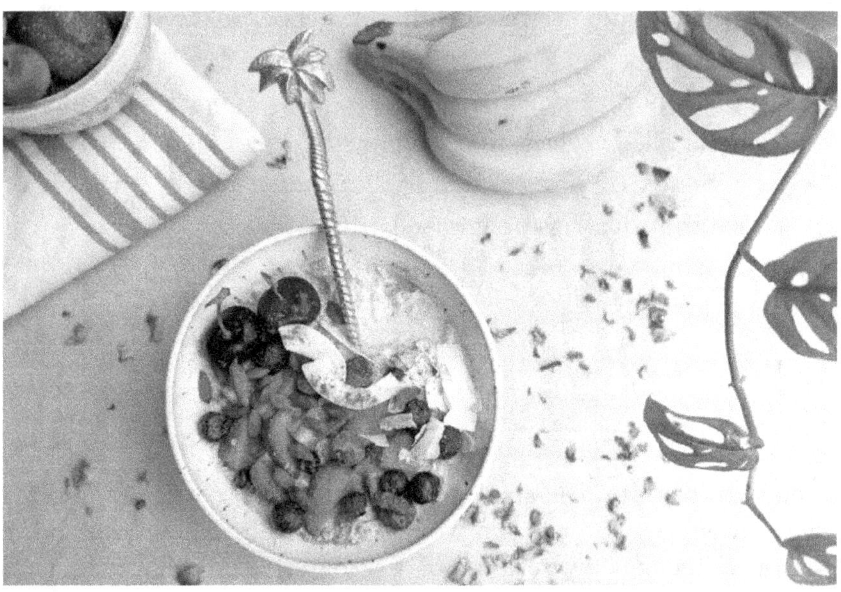

It's the last day! It seems like a week has gone by so fast. How are you feeling now? Wrap up your week with the following dishes then you can make your own meal plan for the next week:

- **Breakfast:** A bowl of whole-grain oats with maple syrup, cinnamon, and dates. Top this with walnuts and blackberries.
- **Lunch:** Two cups of steamed kale leaves with olives, cucumber, tomato, Parmesan cheese, and a drizzle of fresh

lemon juice. Pair this with a portion of grilled oily fish like sardines.

- **Dinner:** One cup of arugula with herbs and a drizzle of lemon juice. Pair this with two boiled artichokes seasoned with salt, pepper, garlic powder, and olive oil.
- **Snack (if you get hungry between meals):** A small serving of Greek yogurt with nuts and honey.

Conclusion:

# Improving Your Life Through Your

# Diet

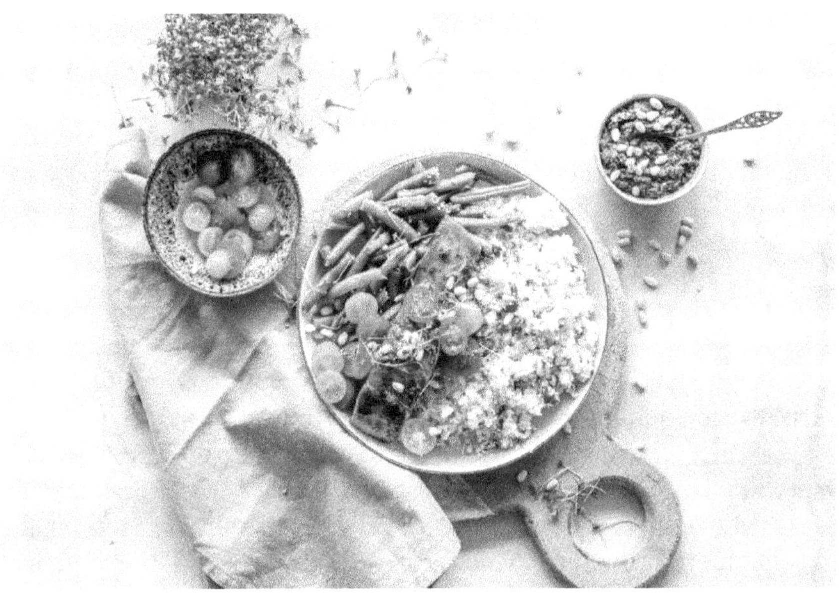

For millennia, the Mediterranean diet has been followed by people all over the world. Over the years, this traditional diet hasn't changed much. Since the beginning, it has been predominantly based on fresh and whole foods like fruits, vegetables, nuts, seeds, olive oil, and fish. Because of how simple and effective it is, the Mediterranean diet has stood the test of time. This style of eating offers a number of health benefits, especially in terms of cardiovascular health.

Combining the pescatarian diet with the Mediterranean diet offers even more benefits as these two diets are similar to each other. This winning combination is called the Pesco-Mediterranean diet and it is considered the ideal diet for long-term health. Adding intermittent fasting to the mix (with a fasting window between 8 to 12 hours) makes things even better for you. This plant-rich diet focuses on fish and seafood as your main animal protein sources, which adds to the benefit of being an ideal cardio-protective diet.

By now, you already know all the basics of the Pesco-Mediterranean diet. With everything you have learned in the different chapters of this book, you can now start creating a plan for how you will start this diet. In this book, we started off by defining the Pesco-Mediterranean diet. We broke down the diet by discussing the pescatarian and Mediterranean diets separately to help you see how similar they are and why they work so well together. In the second chapter, we discussed this ideal diet further by explaining how it works and what science has to say about it. Although relatively new, studies that have been conducted about this diet have shown promising results.

Then in Chapter 3, you learned how to start with this diet by learning the foods to eat, the foods to avoid, and even a couple of tips to help you start. In Chapter 4 to Chapter 7, we focused on the benefits of the foods that belong in this diet—fiber, legumes, whole grains, fish, seafood, nuts, seeds, and healthy fats. Knowing all of these should have given you a better understanding of why this diet is so effective. Then we moved on to Chapter 8 where we discussed other aspects of the Pesco-Mediterranean diet, which are the benefits and the potential risks. And in the final chapter, we added intermittent fasting to the diet to make it even more beneficial.

I even added a bonus chapter for you to help kick-start your planning process. Since meal planning can help you stick with the Pesco-Mediterranean diet until it becomes a permanent part of your life, learning how to make a meal plan will be really helpful for you. As promised at the beginning of this book, I have shared with you everything you need to know about the Pesco-Mediterranean diet. Hopefully, all of this information helps you understand why this is considered the "ideal diet" for long-term health and weight management. Now, all you have to do is to start your own Pesco-Mediterranean diet. Take that all-important first step by creating a plan that is geared towards your health goals. Once you have that plan, then you can begin! This diet will surely improve the quality of your life by leaps and bounds. Good luck on your journey and I hope you achieve all of your health goals by applying everything you have learned here.

# References

Admin. (2020, June 2). *Intro to Mediterranean Foods.* Mediterranean Diet Guru. https://mediterraneandietguru.com/intro-to-mediterranean-foods/

American College of Cardiology. (2020a, September 14). *Pesco-Mediterranean diet, intermittent fasting may lower heart disease risk.* Medical Xpress. https://medicalxpress.com/news/2020-09-pesco-mediterranean-diet-intermittent-fasting-heart.html

American College of Cardiology. (2020b, September 19). *Pesco-Mediterranean Diet, Intermittent Fasting May Lower Heart Disease Risk.* AlphaGalileo. https://www.alphagalileo.org/en-gb/Item-Display/ItemId/197149?returnurl=https://www.alphagalileo.org/en-gb/Item-Display/ItemId/197149

Andrews, R. (2009, January 26). *All about intermittent fasting | Precision Nutrition.* Precision Nutrition. https://www.precisionnutrition.com/all-about-intermittent-fasting

Becco, L. B. (2019, December 23). *Everything You Need to Know About Intermittent Fasting.* Experience Life. https://experiencelife.com/article/everything-you-need-to-know-about-intermittent-fasting/

Becker, D. (2020, September 30). *A Cardiologist on the New Pesco-Mediterranean Diet, and What's Best for Heart Health | Expert Opinion.* Inquirer. https://www.inquirer.com/health/expert-opinions/heart-health-pesco-mediterranean-diet-intermittent-fasting-20200930.html

Berman, R. (n.d.). *Maintain a Healthy Weight with the Mediterranean Diet.* Dummies. https://www.dummies.com/food-drink/special-diets/mediterranean-diet/maintain-a-healthy-weight-with-the-mediterranean-diet/

Bowling, N. (2018, July 24). *12 Best Types of Fish to Eat*. Healthline. https://www.healthline.com/health/food-nutrition/11-best-fish-to-eat

Bruno, A. (2015). *10 of the Healthiest Cooking Oils, Explained*. SELF. https://www.self.com/story/10-of-the-healthiest-cooking-oils-explained

Carroll, C. (2020, February 25). *What Is the Mediterranean Diet?* Verywell Fit. https://www.verywellfit.com/mediterranean-diet-overview-2506730

CBS Boston. (2020, September 15). *Study: Pesco-Mediterranean Diet May Be Ideal For Heart Health*. Msn. https://www.msn.com/en-us/health/nutrition/study-pesco-mediterranean-diet-may-be-ideal-for-heart-health/ar-BB192vp8

Cleveland Clinic. (2020, February 17). *11 Best High-Fiber Foods*. Health Essentials from Cleveland Clinic. https://health.clevelandclinic.org/11-best-high-fiber-foods/

Cook, D. (2018, April 20). *13 Healthiest Beans, Grains & Legumes*. Doug Cook RD. https://www.dougcookrd.com/7-healthiest-grains-pulses/

Cox, C. E. (2020, September 15). *Pesco-Mediterranean Diet Should Be the Gold Standard, Says JACC Review*. TctMD. https://www.tctmd.com/news/pesco-mediterranean-diet-should-be-gold-standard-says-jacc-review

Crichton-Stuart, C. (2018, December 6). *Pescatarian diet: Pros, cons, and what to eat*. Medical News Today. https://www.medicalnewstoday.com/articles/323907

Davis, J. L. (n.d.). *Top 10 Sources of Fiber*. WebMD. https://www.webmd.com/diet/features/top-10-sources-of-fiber

Deakin University. (2020). *Nuts and Seeds.* Better Healthy Channel. https://www.betterhealth.vic.gov.au/health/healthyliving/Nuts-and-seeds

Disabled World. (2018). *Nuts and Seeds: Health and Nutrition Benefits.* Disabled World. https://www.disabled-world.com/fitness/nutrition/nuts-seeds/

Dreisbach, S. (2016, March 11). *10 Amazing Health Benefits of Eating More Fiber.* EatingWell. http://www.eatingwell.com/article/287742/10-amazing-health-benefits-of-eating-more-fiber/

Drillinger, M. (2020, September 16). *Pesco-Mediterranean Diet and Intermittent Fasting Can Help Your Heart.* Healthline. https://www.healthline.com/health-news/a-pesco-mediterranean-diet-and-intermittent-fasting-can-help-your-heart#How-intermittent-fasting-can-help

Esposito, K., Marfella, R., Ciotola, M., Di Palo, C., Giugliano, F., Giugliano, G., D'Armiento, M., D'Andrea, F., & Giugliano, D. (2004). Effect of a Mediterranean-Style Diet on Endothelial Dysfunction and Markers of Vascular Inflammation in the Metabolic Syndrome. *JAMA, 292*(12), 1440. https://doi.org/10.1001/jama.292.12.1440

Estruch, R., Ros, E., Salas-Salvadó, J., Covas, M.-I., Corella, D., Arós, F., Gómez-Gracia, E., Ruiz-Gutiérrez, V., Fiol, M., Lapetra, J., Lamuela-Raventos, R. M., Serra-Majem, L., Pintó, X., Basora, J., Muñoz, M. A., Sorlí, J. V., Martínez, J. A., & Martínez-González, M. A. (2013). Primary Prevention of Cardiovascular Disease with a Mediterranean Diet. *New England Journal of Medicine, 368*(14), 1279–1290. https://doi.org/10.1056/nejmoa1200303

Ettinger, J. (2020, March 4). *The 7 Healthiest Beans, Grains and Legumes.* Naturally Savvy. https://naturallysavvy.com/eat/the-7-healthiest-beans-grains-legumes/

Food Network. (2020). *The Health Benefits of Seafood*. Food Network. https://www.foodnetwork.com/how-to/articles/the-health-benefits-of-seafood

Frey, M. (2019). *What Is a Pescatarian Diet?* Verywell Fit. https://www.verywellfit.com/pescatarian-diet-4174528

Gold, B. (2019, December 5). *These Are the Healthiest Fish and Seafood Varieties*. Real Simple. https://www.realsimple.com/food-recipes/recipe-collections-favorites/healthy-meals/healthiest-seafood

Grains & Legumes Nutrition Council. (2020). *Whole Grains*. Grains & Legumes Nutrition Council. https://www.glnc.org.au/grains/grains-and-nutrition/wholegrains/

Gunnars, K. (2017). *6 Popular Ways to Do Intermittent Fasting*. Healthline. https://www.healthline.com/nutrition/6-ways-to-do-intermittent-fasting

Gunnars, K. (2018a). *22 High-Fiber Foods You Should Eat*. Healthline. https://www.healthline.com/nutrition/22-high-fiber-foods

Gunnars, K. (2018b, May 23). *Why Is Fiber Good for You? The Crunchy Truth*. Healthline. https://www.healthline.com/nutrition/why-is-fiber-good-for-you

Gunnars, K. (2020, January 5). *6 Popular Ways to Do Intermittent Fasting*. EcoWatch. https://www.ecowatch.com/popular-ways-to-do-intermittent-fasting-2644135767.html?rebelltitem=3#rebelltitem3

Harvard T.H. Chan. (2018, December 12). *Diet Review: Mediterranean Diet*. The Nutrition Source. https://www.hsph.harvard.edu/nutritionsource/healthy-weight/diet-reviews/mediterranean-diet/

Health Fitness Revolution. (2015, June 4). *Top 10 Health Benefits of Eating Seafood*. Health Fitness Revolution.

https://www.healthfitnessrevolution.com/top-10-health-benefits-eating-seafood/

Heid, M. (2020, October 1). *Science Might Have Identified the Optimal Human Diet.* Medium. https://elemental.medium.com/science-might-have-identified-the-optimal-human-diet-ec618b2fb8f2

Henderson, E. (2020, September 22). *Pesco-Mediterranean Diet May Lower Risk for Heart Disease.* AZO Life Sciences. https://www.azolifesciences.com/news/20200922/Pesco-Mediterranean-Diet-May-Lower-Risk-for-Heart-Disease.aspx

Jennings, K.-A. (2017, March 10). *What Is a Pescatarian and What Do They Eat?* Healthline. https://www.healthline.com/nutrition/pescatarian-diet

Johnson, J. (2019, January 18). *Mediterranean diet: A guide and 7-day meal plan.* Medical News Today. https://www.medicalnewstoday.com/articles/324221

Johnson, O. (2020, May 23). *Mediterranean Diet Meal Plan For A Smooth-Flowing Weight Loss Journey.* BetterMe. https://betterme.world/articles/mediterranean-diet-meal-plan/

Joseph, M. (2018, August 23). *21 Healthy Types of Seafood: the Best Options.* Nutrition Advance. https://www.nutritionadvance.com/types-of-seafood/

Joseph, T. (2020). *What Are Two Benefits of Eating Oils?* SF Gate. https://healthyeating.sfgate.com/two-benefits-eating-oils-7360.html

Kaur, A. (2018, April 28). *Legumes & Whole Grains Health Benefits | Source of Amino Acids.* Truweight Blog. https://truweight.in/blog/health/legumes-grains-perfect-pairing.html

Kenler, M. (2020, October 26). *The Pescatarian Diet REVIEW | Benefits, Risks, and What to Eat!* Anabolic Aliens. https://www.anabolicaliens.com/blog/the-pescatarian-diet-review

Leech, J. (2019, June 11). *11 Evidence-Based Health Benefits of Eating Fish*. Healthline. https://www.healthline.com/nutrition/11-health-benefits-of-fish

Mahase, E. (2019). Vegetarian and Pescatarian Diets are Linked to Lower Risk of Ischaemic Heart Disease, Study Finds. *BMJ*, l5397. https://doi.org/10.1136/bmj.l5397

Malacoff, J. (2019, February 27). *The 10 Healthiest Nuts and Seeds*. Shape. https://www.shape.com/healthy-eating/diet-tips/healthiest-nuts-and-seeds

Mayo Clinic Staff. (2018). *Dietary Fiber: Essential for a Healthy Diet*. Mayo Clinic. https://www.mayoclinic.org/healthy-lifestyle/nutrition-and-healthy-eating/in-depth/fiber/art-20043983

Mayo Clinic Staff. (2019). *Mediterranean diet: A heart-healthy eating plan*. Mayo Clinic. https://www.mayoclinic.org/healthy-lifestyle/nutrition-and-healthy-eating/in-depth/mediterranean-diet/art-20047801

McNulty, R. (2020, September 17). *Pesco-Mediterranean Diet May Be the Key to a Healthy Heart*. Muscle & Fitness. https://www.muscleandfitness.com/nutrition/healthy-eating/a-pesco-mediterranean-diet-may-be-the-key-to-a-healthy-heart/

Medline Plus. (2013). *Mediterranean diet: MedlinePlus Medical Encyclopedia*. Medline Plus. https://medlineplus.gov/ency/patientinstructions/000110.htm

Migala, J. (2019, April 18). *Going Pescatarian 101: Food List, Meal Plan, Benefits, and More*. EverydayHealth. https://www.everydayhealth.com/diet-nutrition/pescatarian-diet-food-list-meal-plan-benefits-risks-more/

Migala, J. (2020, April 20). *The 7 Types of Intermittent Fasting, and What to Know About Them*. Everyday Health. https://www.everydayhealth.com/diet-nutrition/diet/types-intermittent-fasting-which-best-you/

Moore, A. (2020, September 14). *Study Finds The Pesco-Mediterranean Diet Is Ideal For Cardiovascular Health*. Mind Body Green. https://www.mindbodygreen.com/articles/pesco-mediterranean-diet-heart-health-study

msn. (2019, January 20). *Super Seeds and Nuts You Should Include in Your Diet*. Msn. https://www.msn.com/en-in/foodanddrink/foodnews/super-seeds-and-nuts-you-should-include-in-your-diet/ar-BBJmDw5

Murphy, J. (2020, June 9). *8 healthiest fish to eat, and 4 to avoid*. MDLinx. https://www.mdlinx.com/article/8-healthiest-fish-to-eat-and-4-to-avoid/340eDPcbxPql5dvMWL9vvx

Myupchar. (2020, September 16). *Study Recommends Pesco-Mediterranean Diet Along with Intermittent Fasting for Better Heart Health*. Firstpost. https://www.firstpost.com/health/study-recommends-pesco-mediterranean-diet-along-with-intermittent-fasting-for-better-heart-health-8820611.html

O Brien, P. (2020a, October 13). *Pesco Mediterranean Diet Meals: a Typical Day on a Plate*. KOKO. https://koko.news/eat/Pesco-Mediterranean-diet-meals-a-typical-day-on-a-plate-20201013-0008.html

O Brien, P. (2020b, October 13). *Pesco Mediterranean Diet: The Amazing Benefits of the World's Healthiest Diet*. KOKO. https://koko.news/Ranked-best-for-third-year-in-a-row-benefits-of-the-Mediterranean-diet-t202005190002.html

O'Keefe, J. H., Torres-Acosta, N., O'Keefe, E. L., Saeed, I. M., Lavie, C. J., Smith, S. E., & Ros, E. (2020). A Pesco-Mediterranean Diet With Intermittent Fasting: JACC Review Topic of the Week. *Journal of the American College of Cardiology, 76*(12), 1484–1493. https://doi.org/10.1016/j.jacc.2020.07.049

Pawlowski, A. (2020, September 16). *A Twist on the Mediterranean Diet is "Ideal" for Heart Health, Doctors Declare*. TODAY. https://www.today.com/health/pesco-mediterranean-diet-pescatarian-twist-fish-best-diet-heart-health-t191748

Polak, R., Phillips, E. M., & Campbell, A. (2015). Legumes: Health Benefits and Culinary Approaches to Increase Intake. *Clinical Diabetes, 33*(4), 198–205. https://doi.org/10.2337/diaclin.33.4.198

Raman, R. (2018, July 14). *14 Healthy Whole-Grain Foods (Including Gluten-Free Options).* Healthline. https://www.healthline.com/nutrition/whole-grain-foods

Robertson, R. (2017). *The 9 Healthiest Beans and Legumes You Can Eat.* Healthline. https://www.healthline.com/nutrition/healthiest-beans-legumes

Roston, B. A. (2020, September 14). *Study Finds Modified Mediterranean Diet and Fasting Combo Offers Best Results.* SlashGear. https://www.slashgear.com/study-finds-modified-mediterranean-diet-and-fasting-combo-offers-best-results-14637986/

Rubenfire, M. (2020, September 14). *Pesco-Mediterranean Diet With Intermittent Fasting.* American College of Cardiology. https://www.acc.org/latest-in-cardiology/ten-points-to-remember/2020/09/14/15/38/a-pesco-mediterranean-diet-with-intermittent

Rushlau, K. (2020, September 21). *Review Points to "Pesco-Mediterranean" Diet with Intermittent Fasting for Heart Health.* Integrative Practitioner. https://www.integrativepractitioner.com/nutrition/news/2020-09-21-review-points-to-pesco-mediterranean-diet-with-intermittent-fasting-for-heart-health

Saga. (2019, June 21). *Health benefits of oils: olive, flaxseed, avocado & more - Saga.* Saga. https://www.saga.co.uk/magazine/health-wellbeing/diet-nutrition/nutrition/health-benefits-of-different-oils

Salas-Salvado, J., Bullo, M., Babio, N., Martinez-Gonzalez, M. A., Ibarrola-Jurado, N., Basora, J., Estruch, R., Covas, M. I., Corella, D., Aros, F., Ruiz-Gutierrez, V., & Ros, E. (2010).

Reduction in the Incidence of Type 2 Diabetes With the Mediterranean Diet: Results of the PREDIMED-Reus nutrition intervention randomized trial. *Diabetes Care, 34*(1), 14–19. https://doi.org/10.2337/dc10-1288

*Seafood Nutrition Overview.* (2020). Seafood Health Facts. https://www.seafoodhealthfacts.org/seafood-nutrition/healthcare-professionals/seafood-nutrition-overview

Sifferlin, A. (2018, July 23). *The 10 Best and Worst Oils For Your Health.* Time. https://time.com/5342337/best-worst-cooking-oils-for-your-health/

Springston, J. (2020). *Intermittent Fasting, Pesco-Mediterranean Diet Can Improve Health.* Relias Media. https://www.reliasmedia.com/articles/146951-intermittent-fasting-pesco-mediterranean-diet-can-improve-health

Stillman, J. (2020, October 13). *Scientists Say They Have Zeroed In on the World's Healthiest Diet.* Inc. https://www.inc.com/jessica-stillman/health-productivity-nutrition-diet.html

Vitta, S. (2020, September 15). *Pesco-Mediterranean Diet Reduces Heart Disease Risk.* Medindia. https://www.medindia.net/news/lifestyleandwellness/pesco-mediterranean-diet-reduces-heart-disease-risk-197562-1.htm

Webb, D. (2014). *Beans and Grains: The Perfect Pairing.* Today's Dietitian. https://www.todaysdietitian.com/newarchives/120914p36.shtml

Wozniak, H., Larpin, C., de Mestral, C., Guessous, I., Reny, J.-L., & Stringhini, S. (2020). Vegetarian, Pescatarian, and Flexitarian Diets: Sociodemographic Determinants and Association with Cardiovascular Risk Factors in a Swiss Urban Population. *The British Journal of Nutrition, 124*(8), 844–852. https://doi.org/10.1017/S0007114520001762

Zietsman, G. (2020, September 29). *Study recommends combo of Mediterranean diet and intermittent fasting for the heart.* Health24.

https://m.health24.com/Diet-and-nutrition/Healthy-diets/study-recommends-combo-of-mediterranean-diet-and-intermittent-fasting-for-the-heart-20200929-3

# Image References

All images have been sourced from https://unsplash.com

Figure 1: Healthy Diet. From Unsplash, by Ella Olsson, 2018. https://unsplash.com/photos/rD3YrnhTmf0

Figure 2: Pescatarian Diet. From Unsplash, by Brooke Lark, 2017. https://unsplash.com/photos/C1fMH2Vej8A

Figure 3: Mediterranean Diet. From Unsplash, by Anna Pelzer, 2017. https://unsplash.com/photos/IGfIGP5ONV0

Figure 4: Pesco-Mediterranean Diet. From Unsplash, by Hermes Rivera, 2017. https://unsplash.com/photos/Ww8eQWjMJWk

Figure 5: What to Eat. From Unsplash, by Dan Gold, 2017. https://unsplash.com/photos/4_jhDO54BYg

Figure 6: Starting the Diet. From Unsplash, by Pablo Merchán Montes, 2018. https://unsplash.com/photos/Orz90t6o0e4

Figure 7: Benefits of Fiber. From Unsplash, by Ella Olsson, 2018. https://unsplash.com/photos/7EhPbdAQG-s

Figure 8: Legumes. From Unsplash, by Shelley Pauls, 2019. https://unsplash.com/photos/t4X660oKiYs

Figure 9: Whole Grains. From Unsplash, by Pierre Bamin, 2020. https://unsplash.com/photos/oZ4Krez3X5o

Figure 10: Fish and Seafood. From Unsplash, by Frank Vessia, 2018. https://unsplash.com/photos/RlZsdoTnFCI

Figure 11: Healthy Seafood. From Unsplash, by Louis Hansel, 2019. https://unsplash.com/photos/jZjIAjz_AHE

Figure 12: Benefits of Oils. From Unsplash, by Jessica Lewis, 2018. https://unsplash.com/photos/FVbZZpP58dY